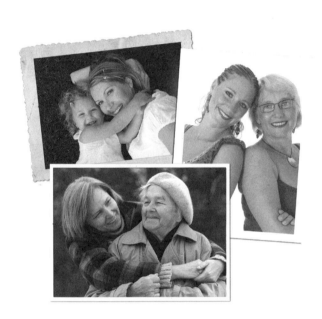

D0927167

My *Mom* Has Alzheimer's

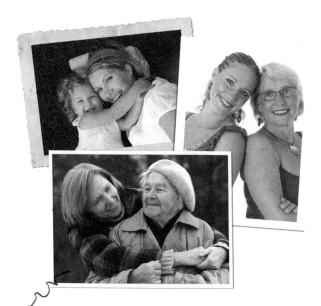

Inspiration and Help for Caregivers

Linda A. Born

Alachua, Florida 32615

Bridge-Logos
Alachua, FL 32615 USA

My Mom Has Alzheimer's
by Linda A. Born

Copyright ©2009 by Bridge-Logos

Printed in the United States of America.

Library of Congress Catalog Card Number: 2009933292
International Standard Book Number 978-0-88270-926-0

Scripture quotations in this book are from the *Holy Bible, New International Version*®. NIV®. Copyright © 1973, 1978, 1984 by International Bible Society. Used by permission of Zondervan. All rights reserved.

Scripture quotations marked MSG are taken from *The Message.* Copyright ©1993, 1994, 1995, 1996, 2000, 2001, 2002. Used by permission of NavPress Publishing Group.

Scripture quotations marked NLT are taken from the *Holy Bible, New Living Translation,* copyright © 1996. Used by permission of Tyndale House Publishers, Inc., Wheaton, Illinois 60189. All rights reserved.

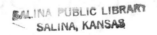

Dedication

To John, my co-caregiver.

Thank you for all the ways you take care of our family.

Contents

Preface

I'd been worried about Mother for quite some time. Perhaps it was the day she called me because she couldn't put the batteries into the T.V. remote.

Or maybe it was the time she had a flat tire on the highway and was unable to use her cell phone to call for help, even though I had taped explicit instructions onto the dashboard of her car.

And then there were the repetitive phrases. She'd get stuck on one adjective or phrase and use it to the exclusion of all other words. For some reason, one of her pet phrases was, and remains, "That'll be a plus." I remember one day when she was justifiably miffed at me for having been rude to her, I said, "I'm going home now, Mom."

"That'll be a plus," she said sincerely.

These behaviors were uncharacteristic. My mother had always been self-sufficient; she was a kind and capable Christian lady who led Bible studies and taught Sunday school. She was a wordsmith, never without an open journal in her lap and pen in hand. She continued to fill journal pages with her thoughts and prayers, but I noticed that she was struggling more to think of words for commonplace objects. The changes were gradual, and I attributed them to the natural aging process.

Finally, there came a late winter afternoon when Mother was telling a story about the woodlot on her father's farm, and she could not think of the word, "stump."

"You know," she said, "… the thing that's left after they chop down the tree."

I had suppressed my worry for months, and for some reason this relatively minor memory glitch brought my fears into sharp focus. Time stopped, my world shifted, and I knew with certainty that something was very wrong. I made a doctor's appointment and spent a few days researching all possible causes for Mom's symptoms of dementia. Perhaps she had suffered mini strokes, maybe her nutrition was inadequate, or she might be suffering from depression. "Anything but Alzheimer's," I thought. I'd always harbored a kind of terror at the thought of the helplessness and hopelessness I associated with this disease. I took my mother to the doctor and after extensive tests we received her diagnosis: dementia of the Alzheimer type.

The devotions in this book came from God's counsel to me as I made the transition from the role of being my mother's beloved daughter to that of her beloved caregiver. The Lord helped me with every stage of this journey: with the anger, the sense of abandonment, the loneliness, grief, and fear. I felt like an orphan, but He said, "I will never leave you or forsake you" (Joshua 1:5). I had never truly accepted or dealt with the certainty of physical death, my own or that of someone I love. God said, "Even though you walk through the valley of the shadow of death, you need fear no evil, for I am with you" (Psalm 23, paraphrased).

We have found to our blessing that God's grace truly is sufficient for every need. If someone you love suffers from dementia, these writings are dedicated to you with love and a prayer that you will be encouraged and blessed.

Because of its wide scope of grief, joy, laughter, and tears, I recommend reading this book as it was written, one entry a day in the form of a devotion. My mother and I offer to you these vignettes from our lives with a prayer that you will share the encouragement and hope that we have received from our blessed Lord.

Introduction

$\mathcal{E}$ach chapter in this devotional book has a special message of hope and encouragement.

Chapter 1: Making the Transition: Caregiving can either be viewed as an interruption in one's life plan or as the fulfillment of a holy purpose ordained by God.

Chapter 2: Facing the Grief: If we do not give voice to the emotion we feel, we rob ourselves of the gift of an awareness of God's compassion.

Chapter 3: Releasing the Bad Stuff: Guilt, resentment, and a critical spirit are caregiving pitfalls, and to love as we have been loved and forgive as we have been forgiven require God's grace.

Chapter 4: Honor and Respect: To respond in love to unlovable behaviors entails more than mere silence; Jesus' response to persecution was to commit an act of love through His death on the Cross.

Chapter 5: Abide in the Lord: We can't control the workings of the loom that weaves the fabric of our lives, but we can influence the color and pattern that is visible to mortal eyes as we abide and obey.

Chapter 6: You Might As Well Laugh: Laughter prevents the perspective of both caregiver and patient from becoming unbearably grim.

Chapter 7: A Network of Support: Medical expertise, legal counsel and respite care are important services for caregivers, but the central pillar of strength is an abiding relationship with the Lord.

Chapter 8: Hold to Hope: In difficult times we are to remember the Lord, praise His name, and entrust ourselves into God's hands.

Chapter 9: Beautiful in Each Season: Quotes from my mother offer a fascinating window into the cognitive processes of an Alzheimer patient, and the peace afforded by a deep faith in God even as she loses the capability to think and reason logically.

Chapter 10: Death to Life: Jesus Christ has conquered death; His purpose in coming was to deliver us and set us free; He is trustworthy, and He is in control.

Chapter 11: Questions and Answers: Caregivers must learn to respond to negative behaviors from a clinical rather than an emotional perspective. It is a difficult transition, made easier by the recognition that although the rules of the relationship change, love remains.

Chapter One

Making the Transition

An important understanding is that lifelong roles were not replaced with new identities. Instead, we added the titles of "caregiver" and "patient", as though we had earned new degrees in the school of life. We had been mother and daughter, now we were mother/patient and daughter/caregiver.

—Linda

Just remember, I'm still your mother.

—Anna Ruth

Day 1

Maintain What Remains

A diagnosis of Alzheimer's is frightening, to say the least.
Don't allow yourself to be paralyzed by fear—
God is with you.

One morning soon after my mother had been diagnosed with Alzheimer's disease, my daily Bible reading was from 2 Kings, chapter 18. In verses 28 through 36, a field commander from the enemy taunts the Hebrew people saying, "Has anyone ever escaped from the hand of the king of Assyria?"

And the people are disheartened and remain silent.

When my mother was diagnosed with Alzheimer's, I responded much as the Hebrew people did to the words spoken by the enemy commander. No one recovers from Alzheimer's. In face of this fact, I remained silent. I did not pray much at all for my mother's cognitive health. I took care of her physical needs, and I prayed for her emotional well being, but initially I did not pray regarding the disease that had been projected to cause increasing devastation in her brain.

I came to understand that I could pray very specifically for my mother's health, with the Holy Spirit's guidance. It was not in my heart to pray for healing, but rather, to focus on maintenance. I recognized that it was not yet time to begin a deathwatch. We could work hard to maintain what remained.

Today's Scripture: *"Therefore, pray for the remnant that still survives" (2 Kings 19:4b). "Do not be afraid of what you have heard" (2 Kings 19:6b).*

Caregiving Strategies:

• Play games with your loved one that have been enjoyed in the past, but don't attempt to teach a new game.

• Take the initiative to help your loved one to stay in contact with friends—telephone calls are perfect because they are generally of short duration.

• Be proactive in planning for adequate hydration, nutrition and exercise.

• Ask and keep asking others to pray for your loved one *and* for you.

Day 2

Life Interruption or Life Purpose?

*A*s I began caregiving duties for my mother, I felt a suffocating sensation of stress that came more from a feeling that I should have been elsewhere than from any true crunch for time. I had been able to cut my teaching job to half days in order to spend more time with Mom. My mornings legitimately belonged to her, and yet as I completed each day's chores in Mom's apartment I felt wound tight, as though I were late to a meeting or ought to have been doing something else. There was no joy for me in the routine chores involved in making life pleasant for Mom.

One morning during my devotion time, a question came to mind, "What is your purpose in life?"

"Ok, I know the answer to this one," I thought. "My purpose in life is to give praise, glory, and honor to God." I waited confidently for the Lord's smile of approval, but I did not feel the warmth of His endorsement of my pat answer. As I waited before Him, it came to me that one of the most important ministries ordained for me in this life is to care for my mother. This interlude that I had seen as an interruption in my life's plan was in fact, a fulfillment of a holy purpose assigned to me by God.

5

God allows our lives to mirror that perfect life of Jesus Christ. Jesus willingly gave His life for us. He did it out of obedience and love, and for additional reasons that I can't comprehend because I am not sufficiently like Him to see clearly with His perspective. In caring for my mother, I had the opportunity to lay down my life for Him by allowing His sacrificial love to flow through me to Mom. Instead, I had come perilously close to self-pity. I had kept my mouth tightly closed while ministering to Mom, only then to release the pent up frustration by being rude to my husband. I found that I had given way to resentment toward my mother for interrupting what I had seen to be my life's plan. This robbed me of the ability to minister in love and acceptance toward her.

I remembered when I began my career as a teacher that I had experienced such a strong sense of mission and of being exactly where I was supposed to be. I sensed now that the Lord desired me to have that same kind of commitment in this new ministry of caring for Mom.

Caregiver's Prayer

Father, please grant us as caregivers the grace to accept the truth that this time of service is a part of your holy purpose for our lives. Bring to us a sense of mission and the understanding that you have placed this time before us as an opportunity to serve. Amen.

Today's Scripture: *"Whatever you do, do it all for the glory of God"* (1 Corinthians 10:31).

Day 3

Get Up From There and Be My Mother!

Not long after Mom came to live with us, I suffered a case of influenza and had to go to bed for nearly a week. I had always believed that if I became ill or disabled that I would be the recipient of empathy, sympathy, and love. Well-meaning friends did indeed shower me with phone calls and questions about my well-being, but my husband and son seemed oddly distant, although they both willingly completed extra household tasks. I express love to my family through acts of service, and regardless of the legitimacy of my illness, the end result was that my guys were not receiving their usual quota of tender loving care. They were genuinely worried about me, but they also felt abandoned because I was not looking after them as I usually did, and in fact, I needed them to take care of me. My then seventeen-year-old son Jonathan, who is normally a kind and empathetic young man, acted oblivious to any change in my level of functioning while my husband was completely silent as he took over a portion of the chores I usually did. He worked quickly and bore an air of harried stress. He avoided eye contact with me altogether. It was uncomfortable for me to recognize that this was exactly how I had been acting toward my mother.

I certainly did not rain down flowers and chocolates on my mother's head as she began to manifest the symptoms of Alzheimer's. I had depended on her to be the one person in my world who could be trusted to drop everything and rush to my side in any crisis large or small. When she became disabled I felt that she'd let me down, and I was silently resentful. I felt that this new role reversal was a travesty, and although I did not demand that she get out of her chair and minister to *my* needs, in my heart I felt that such a request would have been justified. I slowly came to accept the changes in my mother's level of functioning, but it took time. In my temporary infirmity I recognized the need to extend to my loved ones the same grace that had been given me.

Today's Scripture: *"Bear with each other and forgive whatever grievances you may have against one another. Forgive as the Lord forgave you" (Colossians 3:13).*

Insight: I had to suffer an illness myself in order to empathize with my mother's decreased level of functioning. Perhaps you can learn from my experience so that the Lord doesn't have to bless you with temporary infirmity! Our loved ones can't help having fallen prey to dementia any more than I could help not being able to perform my usual chores while suffering from the flu.

Day 4

Don't Just Face the Facts—Face Jesus!

One day a friend stopped me in the hallway of the school where we both work. She wanted to tell me that her mother had been diagnosed with Alzheimer's disease. Both of us were fighting tears as I put my arms around her in sympathy. The next day I placed a sheaf of handouts into her trembling hands: pages full of information about caregiving, the stages of the disease, and symptoms one might expect to observe. However, I looked her in the eye and said, "Educate yourself, *but* don't let this information become your foundation of what is truth. The Lord is the only one who knows the future." I wanted her to share my conviction that God intends us good and not harm, and that He will make a way for us through any difficulty.

When my mother was first diagnosed with Alzheimer's, I set out to educate myself about the disease. I am a person who wants to understand how things of the mind, body, and spirit work, and I turned this thirst for knowledge and understanding to my investigation of this malady that had robbed my mother of her ability to function independently.

The predictions were not pleasant. They also have not yet developed. When my mother began medication, she experienced an improvement that has been maintained for four years at this writing. There are not many positive aspects to a diagnosis of Alzheimer's, but the fact that it is many times a slow progressing disease can grant a blessed oasis of time in which to adjust, adapt, and accept.

None of us know the day, hour, or minute when we will be called home. God is sovereign over life, death, and everything between. There is great peace in accepting this fact. "In his heart a man plans his course, but the LORD determines his steps" (Proverbs 16:9).

Oswald Chambers asks us, "Can you trust Jesus Christ where your common sense cannot trust Him?" Common sense based upon the facts of the expected progression of Alzheimer's disease will lead to despair. Faith based upon the reality of Jesus Christ offers hope.[1]

Insight: When well-meaning friends begin to make dire predictions for the future, do not listen, and don't go there yourself. The future is in God's hands, and you can trust Him. No one but the Lord knows the future. Follow Him in your present and leave tomorrow in His hands.

Day 5

Zechariah and Doubt

J have always had empathy for Zechariah. I'm talking about Zechariah of the New Testament, the father of John the Baptist. You'll remember that Zechariah was stricken dumb for speaking doubtfully to the angel Gabriel about the holy events foretold.

Scripture tells of how the Holy Spirit came upon Zechariah, and I imagine that I can see evidence of his life's heart-hurts in his song (See Luke 1:67-80.) Those hurts mirror my own heart's cries as I've struggled with the results of my mother's dementia.

Zechariah rejoices in redemption—*perhaps he had felt trapped in the circumstances of his life.*

He praised God for the strength of salvation in the Messiah who was to come—*perhaps he had been weak.*

He speaks with joy of the fulfillment of prophesies—*his heart might have grown cold with waiting and watching.*

He speaks of rescue from the hands of enemies—*it is possible that in Zechariah's service for God there had been critics and judges.*

He says that this rescue would, "Enable us to serve Him without fear" (Luke 1:74)—*maybe Zechariah had been afraid of the future.*

Zechariah says that now Israel would be able to serve God, "In holiness and righteousness before Him all our days" (Luke 1:75)—*perhaps he had distrusted himself and his own motives, and had feared that sins of bitterness of heart over his life's circumstances would rob him of holiness and righteousness before the Lord.*

The Lord disciplined Zechariah, but He heard his heart cries and blessed him nevertheless. Zechariah lived to see the fulfillment of a holy promise given him by God. You and I can cling to the fulfillment of God's promise given us in Jesus Christ.

Today's Scripture: *"Because of God's tender mercy, the morning light from heaven is about to break upon us, to give light to those who sit in darkness and in the shadow of death, and to guide us to the path of peace" (Luke 1:78-79, NLT).*

Day 6

A Pet for Mom

*B*efore my mother moved into our home, I researched ways to help her to make the transition successfully. Various resources told me that a pet is good therapy for Alzheimer patients. I was not enthusiastic. Pets shed and make messes that have to be cleaned up. I was fairly certain that fulfilling my new role as "Alzheimer Caregiver" was going to be about all I could handle. It did not seem prudent to add the title of pet owner to my rapidly lengthening list of job descriptions. However, for my mother's sake, I began to consider the adoption of a cat or a dog. After much collaboration with friends and relatives, I came to the conclusion that a declawed, short-haired, cat would be the best option for us. I prayed that if God really wanted us to have a cat that He would provide one, and I specifically requested not to have to deal with a kitten (bah, humbug). Feeling safe from feline intrusion, I put the issue out of my mind.

Two days later a friend called to ask whether we would like to have her mother's cat. Her mother, who also had Alzheimer's, could no longer care for the animal. Enter Poky, a seven-year-old female Alzheimer's Care Cat with experience.

Mom was not pleased. "I do not want that cat on my lap," she said. And she meant it. Being dumped onto the floor immediately after she had the temerity to leap into my mother's lap did not daunt Poky. This happened about twenty times a day during the first week of her residence with us. Between rejections Poky would unconcernedly groom her sleek, gray coat. She would then laze on the floor, green eyes focused appraisingly upon Mother's face.

I returned home from work one day to find Poky ensconced upon Mother's lap, purring. With no hint of her previous aversion Mother said, "You know, this is a beautiful cat. We are friends." Having claimed Mom as her own, Poky was in the mood to conquer new territory. She leaped gracefully to the floor and strolled over to me. To Mother's chagrin, Poky jumped into my lap and lay down.

"That cat," Mother said, "is fickle."

Poky was a comfort to my mother and provided her with much needed companionship. An unexpected bonus was the enjoyment she brought to each member of our family.

Caregiver's Prayer

Father, help me as a caregiver to be open to your nudges to provide creative solutions to the difficulties that my loved ones face. In Jesus' name I pray, Amen.

Day 7

Beauty in Nature Reveals God

There was a mile long stretch of country road that I drove each day as I traveled to the school where I worked. It was a straight line that made a white, dusty diameter across a ring of pastures and fields. With the dome of sky stretching down to meet the horizon in a perfect circle around me, it was like being contained in the landscape of a huge snow globe. Most winters we had snow enough to bring that fantasy to life, but in the spring the illusion continued as white tufts from cottonwood trees filled the air. During this daily drive I learned that taking a moment to appreciate the beauty of God's creation refreshes the soul.

In the early days of Mom's time with us in our home, we often found ourselves at odds with one another. She felt confused and threatened by the change in her surroundings, and I was weary from the increased workload and from worriment. We could, however, come to a place of harmony during our late afternoon walks. No matter what ill-tempered words had passed between us, once we stepped outside and filled our eyes with the beauty of the sky and landscape, the mood lightened. "Oooh look at those clouds, just look at them," Mom would exclaim. Or, "Look at the moon! Look at the evening star!" As I looked and ooohed and aaahed along with my mother, we found peace at the common ground of appreciation for God's provision of loveliness for us.

Scripture reveals the reason that beauty in nature grants such peace. "For since the creation of the world God's invisible qualities—His eternal power and divine nature—have been clearly seen, being understood from what has been made" (Romans 1:20). Our God is invisible, but He has revealed much of himself to us in creation. During stress-filled days it is especially important to take time to appreciate the beauty of nature. Just as viewing an artist's work reveals something to us of the artist's character, creation reveals the Creator.

Today's Scripture: *"He leads me beside quiet waters, He restores my soul" (Psalm 23:2-3).*

Caregiving Strategy

Find time to enjoy the beauty of God's creation with your loved one.

Day 8

Looking at Mom Through God's Eyes

My husband's grandmother lived in a nursing home the last few years of her life. One day as I was leaving the facility after a visit with her, I had to wait at the exit because a man and his elderly mother were blocking the door. I stepped back and perused some photos posted on the wall, but I couldn't help overhearing their conversation. He was struggling to reason with his mother over some issue that had left the lady feeling that she had been treated unjustly. She was frail and in a wheelchair, but her grip on his arm was strong and her voice was loud. She berated him at length and finally a nurse came and talked with her. The man told his mother goodbye, promised to return the next day, and the nurse wheeled her away. As I once again approached the door the man turned to me and said, "You know, I have just realized that my mother never was a very nice person."

At the time, my sympathies were all with the poor old lady, who, against her will, had been wheeled back to a room shared with another elderly woman. "Of course she is angry," I thought. "She feels helpless, out of control, frightened and confused, and she has no power to change her circumstances." I felt critical of the son. It was as though up to that moment he had held his mother in high esteem, but that he had dismissed all that she had been because of what she had become.

Now that I have become the caregiver of an elderly parent, my opinion of that troubled man has softened. It is difficult to avoid drawing unfair connections between my mother's present behaviors and the childish anger I felt toward her while I was growing up. For example, one day I overheard my mother threatening to inflict corporal punishment upon the cat, who had knocked an ornament from the Christmas tree.

"If you don't stop that, Kitty," she said, "I'm going to spank you. You wouldn't like that would you?" The words and intonations were identical to those I'd heard many times as a child, and I felt again the sense of injustice I must have suffered over some long ago circumstance when I was sure that I'd been punished unfairly. I was surprised at the sense of outrage I felt because my mother had made what I knew to be a completely harmless threat to an unruly pet. A six-year-old child's emotions resurrected in the mind of a fifty-year-old can result in ridiculous reactions to minor transgressions, and I was grateful that this time I was able to keep from giving voice to my feelings.

We tend to view the past through the lens of the present. It is human nature to shake a fist toward God when our circumstances are painful; Jonah was angry enough to die when God provided the worm that robbed him of the shade of the vine. He was not grateful for the protection the vine had provided him while he sat in its shelter; he was only angry that he'd been deprived of its comfort. (See Jonah 4:1-3.)

Having lived and thrived in the shelter of my mother's nurturing love, I prayed for grace to remember the ease that her work and sacrifice provided for me for so many years.

Caregiver's Prayer

Lord, please guard my perceptions, my reactions, and my words. Please don't allow the trials that my loved one's age and illness cause in the present to rob me of the remembrance of the blessings of the past. Grant me the grace to view my loved one through your eyes. Amen.

Day 9

Love Remains

As soon as my mother was tagged with the label *Alzheimer's disease*, I began to grieve her loss. I transitioned through several stages of understanding in those early weeks and months. At first a terrible pity infused tender compassion and pathos into all of my interactions with Mother. It was as though I was attempting to endure the intense emotion of a funeral visitation for weeks on end, and I couldn't sustain the effort.

I then gave up the grief for anger. In a classic blame the victim state of mind I looked for things my mother had done or failed to do that caused her to fall prey to disease. In the past, my mother performed many roles in my life as she babysat for my children, acted as my confidante and counselor, bought clothes and gifts for me and gloried in my achievements. All of those services came to a halt when dementia struck, and I felt abandoned. My anger expressed itself through a peevish, snappish, demeanor that left mother feeling puzzled and hurt while I drowned in guilt.

I had to make a beginning toward acceptance of who my mother had become, and to release the mother she had been. This release was a process and not an event, and it required moving further into an abiding relationship with

20

God as well as seeking out the support of prayer partners and friends.

Alzheimer's robbed my mother of the capacity to do and remember, not of the ability to feel and to love. At a meeting of an Alzheimer's support group, one woman said that the awareness of loving and being loved is maintained until the end of life, no matter how advanced the dementia. What comfort! I loved my mother selfishly when I loved her for what she could do for me. Now my love had an opportunity to be more Christlike. Furthermore, there was great comfort in the knowledge that my mother was still present and that we still had the opportunity to love one another.

Today's Scripture: *"And now these three remain: faith, hope and love. But the greatest of these is love" (1 Corinthians 13:13).*

Caregiver's Prayer

Father, as caregivers we carry heartbreakingly heavy loads. We pray that you lighten our burdens, send us help, and enable us to stay free of energy draining emotions of bitterness, anger, and resentment. Enable us to release to you those things that cause us pain, provide us healing, and help us to effectively express your love. In Jesus' name we pray, Amen.

Day 10

Less Than Lucid Moments

I became comfortable with the knowledge that despite the changes in her level of functioning, the woman I had known as *Mother* had not been spirited away only to be replaced by a new individual labeled, *Alzheimer patient.* She was still my mom. She had challenges to face, but her personality remained mostly intact as she continued to delight me with her humor and unexpectedly accurate commentaries on her situation.

One day I went into her room and found her with a look of bewilderment on her face. "Linda," she said slowly, "Tell me again why I am here. I mean, I know that this is my furniture, and that you live out in the big part of the house. But why did I move here?"

"Oh boy," I thought to myself. Aloud I said, "Well, Mama, you have Alzheimer's disease, and couldn't fix your own meals or drive anymore, and so we moved you out here where I can take care of you."

A look of relief flooded her face and she snapped her fingers, "Oh, Alzheimer's. Well thank you, that explains it." She picked up her notebook and wrote in large print, "I have Alzheimer's." Then she reached for a book and contentedly began to read.

I was unnerved; because each new sign of my mother's diminishing cognitive function depressed and upset me. After she had gone to bed I came in to check on her and asked tentatively, "Are you ok? Do you know where you are?"

She giggled, "Yes, I know I'm in my apartment, attached to your house, tucked in safe and sound."

I felt silly and said, "Well, earlier you were concerned about why you were here."

She laughed again and said calmly, "I admit that I have my less than lucid moments."

That evening, my mother's attitude and her calm acceptance of her situation were a comfort to me.

Today's Scripture: *"Praise be to the God and Father of our Lord Jesus Christ, the Father of compassion and the God of all comfort, who comforts us in all our troubles, so that we can comfort those in any trouble with the comfort we ourselves have received from God" (2 Corinthians 1:3-4).*

Caregiving Strategy

When in the throes of anger or grief, we might feel it appropriate to explain to the poor dementia patient *the hard facts* of the situation, but as caregivers we must be willing to allow our charges to maintain a blessed ignorance. It is actually a great comfort to recognize that our loved ones who suffer dementia are not aware of the pathos of their circumstances.

Chapter Two

Facing the Grief

I found that merely allowing myself to acknowledge the pain
was not enough. Jesus wanted to bear my grief.
I had to learn to cast my cares on Him.

—Linda

It comes to me it is time for praising my Lord for peace and
comfort, rather than thinking sad thoughts about being alone.

—Anna Ruth

Day 1

Don't Avoid the Lord

The year my mother was diagnosed with Alzheimer's, our daughter was married to a wonderful, Christ-centered man. Despite my joy in their union, I had a difficult time with that transition. I was finally able to admit that I was harboring the secret fear that if my daughter needed me less than she had during her growing up years, then she would love me less. In a sense, I found the opposite to be true. The mature heart filled with the love of Christ as Savior does not need to cling to mere human love, and love free of need is a closer approximation of Christlike love.

I came to recognize that if my daughter had difficulties beyond how to cook a pot roast or what cleaner to use on the bathtub, that I was no longer the key designed for that particular lock. She had outgrown me. All mentor/child relationships are temporary—the child grows up. The fact that my daughter no longer required me for sustenance was not a reason for grief, but rather, an indication that I had done my job well. Because of my close emotional tie to her, this was also a gift and a blessing. I was free of my responsibility for her; free to enjoy her.

Life is full of transitions, and most of us don't like this fact. We would prefer to attain a place of comfort and safety and clutch it to our hearts to keep, but we are not allowed to do so. Just as ocean tides ebb and flow, our lives are always in motion.

Despite the fact that I believed all of the truths I've outlined here, for a time my daughter's leave-taking left a terrible feeling of emptiness in my life. I clutched that emptiness to my heart and tried to rise above it on my own, because I had fallen to the deception that to come to the Lord would necessitate my facing the whole of my grief and pain. I had no desire to hurt more than I hurt already. I finally recognized the fallacy of the idea that God would require my heart to be ripped open and the contents emptied in order for me to gain access to Him. This lie was the enemy's attempt to keep me from the solace that was rightfully mine in the Lord.

These days the lock my key fits perfectly is that of *Alzheimer caregiver*, but this role is also temporary. I pray that when my job as my mother's caregiver comes to an end that I will bring my heavy burden of grief to the Lord quickly and willingly. He has promised that those who mourn shall be comforted, and I pray to avail myself of that comfort.

Today's Scripture: *"There is no one like the God of Jeshurun, who rides on the heavens to help you and on the clouds in His majesty. The eternal God is your refuge, and underneath are the everlasting arms" (Deuteronomy 33:26-27a).*

Insight: Anchor your heart to the Lord. Although everything around you may be in a state of upheaval, God does not change.

Day 2

Cry Out

*W*hen I was sixteen, my family and I moved from a suburb of a fair sized city to a very small town. My sophomore year of high school had been spent as one of hundreds of other tenth graders in a school so large that I had felt insignificant and unnoticed. In my new school, I entered a junior class of just twenty-one members, and found myself the center of attention as *the new girl*. To have so many people pay attention to me and to actually court my favor was a completely novel sensation, and I'm sorry to say that I let it go to my head. I had always been somewhat introverted and sensitive, but under the heady influence of this new popularity, I laughed too loudly and flirted outrageously. I was given the keys to my parents' car, and I drove recklessly. I was having the time of my life, but it all came to a rather predictable end. I soon found myself in an awkward situation involving some adults who had justifiably formed negative opinions of me. Several adolescent boys were angry and hurt because of me, and most frighteningly, a whole contingent of teenage girls did not appreciate the upset I'd caused in the delicate balance of the social hierarchy of their school.

In the middle of a mess I'd made myself, I cried out to the Lord. I wept bitter tears out of the intense agony that comes when an untested heart is injured for the first time. I called out to my Savior to help me, and I was amazed when circumstances turned to my favor almost overnight. Through this small trial, I gained a fledgling knowledge of the fact that my heart could move the heart of God. This was possible, not because of any worthiness on my part, but because of what Christ had done for me through the compassion and love of God, by the power of the Holy Spirit. My only role in my own rescue was to cry out, and because I'd been saved by His grace through the blood of Jesus Christ, God heard my cry.

Over the years my faith in the Lord strengthened each time I cried out to Him and saw rich evidence that He always heard and answered my prayers; not always as I would have wished, but always according to His love. God cannot be manipulated, but His heart can be moved toward us because of His love for us. If we do not give voice to the emotion we feel, we rob ourselves of the gift of an awareness of God's great compassion and love.

Today's Scripture: *"For He will deliver the needy who cry out, the afflicted who have no one to help" (Psalm 72:12). "I cry out to God Most High, to God, {who fulfills} His purpose for me" (Psalm 57:2).*

Insight: Watching someone you love suffer from dementia hurts. Cry out to God with the pain of it, release to Him the whole of it, and rest in the knowledge that He has control of it.

Day 3

Strength for that Long Goodbye

*I*t is said that Alzheimer's disease is a long goodbye, and I learned the truth of this statement. I knew that I was weak, and I knew that I needed to avail myself of the Lord's strength, but exactly how did this appropriation of holy help occur? Examples from Scripture and from a few lessons I learned by doing things the wrong way gave me guidance for the following strength building strategies:

When Daniel fell to the ground, drained of all strength, the Lord touched him and spoke to him, and he was strengthened to stand (See Daniel 10:8-11.) God touches our hearts as we praise Him, and He speaks to us through His Word. *Do not neglect to praise God daily, and to read and meditate upon His Word.*

A search of the New International Version of the Bible revealed that the phrases "fear not," "do not fear," and "do not be afraid," occur for a combined total of 84 times in God's word. *Fear drains strength. Confess your fears to God and profess your faith in Him to provide for you.*

Alzheimer's is a marathon. I found that I could not expect to make it through this testing time in the same way I had sprinted through previous trials of shorter duration; sleeping too little, eating too much, and neglecting to exercise. I was forced to give attention to my physical well being. *As a caregiver, do not neglect your own physical health.*

During the first year of caregiving, I was very nearly overwhelmed by grief and fear. I was greatly helped when a friend invited me to attend a Bible Study with her. The prayer, fellowship, and hugs we exchanged helped more than I can express. *Don't become a loner. Reach out to others. Pray for others and ask them to pray for you.*

Nothing blocked my prayers for strength and help so effectively as disobedience. *Do an obedience check.*

Today's Scripture: *"The Lord will guide you always; He will satisfy your needs in a sun-scorched land and will strengthen your frame" (Isaiah 58:11).*

Day 4

Remembering Lydia

I came into Mom's room one afternoon and found her looking troubled. She thrust a scrap of paper into my hands and said, "Here, could this be done up for the members of the family?"

On the crumpled paper Mom had written, "For Lydia, dear friend and neighbor, for this friendship I have been grateful."

I had known Lydia Jones all my life. Mom and Lydia had developed a friendship nearly fifty years earlier when they were country neighbors in a rural neighborhood. Lydia was the quintessential farm wife, sewing her own clothes, feeding her family from the garden she raised, and gathering friends and neighbors around her table for meals that satisfied body and soul. Our family was often among those Lydia and her husband, Ben, invited into their home, and she became woven into my memory as a dependable and comforting part of my childhood.

I was puzzled by the note and said, "But Mom, Lydia is still alive."

"Then why did I write that?" asked Mom.

We stared at one another and then realization dawned. "I don't know," I said, "unless you got a phone call."

I rummaged on Mom's tabletop and uncovered her notebook from the stack of books and papers scattered there. Sure enough, I found a scribbled note, "Lydia Jones' granddaughter called ... Lydia passed away this morning ... pneumonia, strokes...."

I made phone calls and verified the information. I then called a florist and stressed the clerk's patience by insisting that she include my mother's message, in its entirety, on the card for the family.

Later in the evening I was chatting to my daughter, when tears came to my eyes and I began to tremble. "I'm having some kind of an episode," I joked.

But as the tears began to flow, I recognized the source of my grief. I cried like a lost child over the fact that Lydia Jones was no longer in this world. "This is so strange," I said. "Of course I'm sorry Lydia's gone, and I pray for her family in their loss of a wonderful mother and grandmother, but she hasn't been a part of my life for years. What is the matter with me?"

"Don't you think, Mom," my daughter said gently, "that this taps your grief over Grandma?"

Well, yes. I felt the awful, gut wrenching homesickness I had sometimes experienced as a child when I'd spent a night away from home. Years later, as a supposedly mature adult, I found myself longing for my mother and father and my childhood home once again. I felt surprise at the intensity of the sorrow, as though I'd become sick once again from a disease to which I thought I'd gained immunity.

Apart from the Lord, there would be nothing to do with grief of this caliber but to attempt to bury it. It is too unpleasant to cope with for long; but as I looked toward Jesus I heaved a sigh of relief. "Oh yes, Lord, for a moment

I forgot, but now that I look at you I see that everything is going to be all right."

I was reminded of the truth that I must not bury grief or pain. The admonition to *face it now or face it later* is accurate. When I fail to cry out to the Lord when my heart is hurting, I rob myself of the opportunity to receive His compassion and His love. God is mighty to act on behalf of those who cry out to Him. I must avail myself of the healing balm of Gilead. Expressing pain and grief won't kill me—but *repressing* it just might.

Today's Scripture: *"To comfort all who mourn, and provide for those who grieve in Zion—to bestow on them a crown of beauty instead of ashes, the oil of gladness instead of mourning, and a garment of praise instead of a spirit of despair"* *(Isaiah 61:2b-3a).*

Day 5

I Am Not Alone

There were days when despite all my brave words about drawing on God's strength and releasing the pain, I felt lonely and in grief.

One of those very bad days occurred when, on the advice of the elder law attorney, we purchased a prepaid burial plan for Mom.* This required me to write my mother's obituary and to select a casket.

This was a difficult ordeal. It reminded me of times when I had suffered through a terrible virus. In the midst of it I'd known that the symptoms would soon recede and I would feel better—but right at the point of greatest discomfort the condition seemed permanent. Logically, I knew that there would be life for me after my mother's battle with Alzheimer's was done, but on the evening of the day that I wrote my mother's obituary, it didn't seem so. I could not imagine a life without my mother, without Alzheimer's, and without the heavy heart I had that terrible night.

I came home from that difficult meeting with the funeral home personnel feeling as though my mother was gone already, but I walked through the door and was greeted by her cheerful smile. Later in the evening I found a letter she'd written to her brother reminiscing about their childhood.

It was a wonderfully written letter. I was amazed at how someone who no longer remembered how to make coffee or adjust the radio dials could still write so eloquently. Words had always been my mother's forte.

I took a deep breath and let some of the darkness of the day fall from me. Although putting my mother's affairs in proper order required that I make the arrangements for her funeral ahead of time, she was still with me, and that night I was particularly grateful to have the opportunity for a long goodbye.

Jesus was a man of sorrows, acquainted with grief. We have a Savior who understands our hurt and who will walk through every grief with us.

Today's Scripture: *"The LORD is close to the brokenhearted, and saves those who are crushed in spirit" (Psalm 34:18).*

* Recent legal advice indicates the necessity for caution in purchasing prepaid burial plans and suggests alternate ways of saving for this expense. Our solution was right for us, but please consult your lawyer for professional counsel regarding this important matter.

Day 6

Staying in Balance

Taking care of Mom was a balancing act. I felt as though I was walking a narrow beam labeled *GODLY AND LOVING CAREGIVING BEHAVIORS*, and was constantly in danger of falling off. On one side was the hazard of hardening my heart to my mother's situation so that I didn't have to feel grief over her or fear for my own future. When I fell off on this side of the beam, I became callous and tended to blame Mom for having become infirm. On the other side was overwhelming pathos and grief over the so-called tragedy of Alzheimer's. When I erred to this side I felt anguish of spirit, terrible pity for my mother, grief over losing her, guilt, and a hopelessness that was not of the Lord. There is a legitimate grief that I've written about in tomorrow's devotion, but this was an unholy grief that blinded me to the fact that God was in control and had provided richly for us.

One day when I had fallen to the side of grief and guilt, I served my mother her lunch with an attitude of over-solicitousness and sorrow that must have made her feel that death was imminent. Later, when I opened my journal and began devotions, the Lord brought to mind the time our little dog had gotten his leg injured in a brief but violent encounter with a larger dog. When it was over he limped toward me, and I was so distraught that I burst into tears on his behalf as I stroked his head. When he heard my distress, he put his nose to the air and howled. Just a bit later my husband noticed that he was still limping—but our pup had gotten a bit confused—he was bearing weight on the injured leg and was carrying the opposite paw high in the air while gazing at me piteously. As my devotion time came to a close, I recognized that just as my negative attitude had communicated itself to our little dog, that as a caregiver my negative demeanor could impart fear and grief to my mom.

The sensations of hopelessness felt by a Christian are quickly laid to rest when we look at our Savior's face. Our hearts do not become hard, and we do not fear the grief of dying and death because we know we don't have to bear grievous events alone. Our grief is temporary, but oh the tragedy of hopelessness suffered by those who do not know Christ, or who have refused Him. Now, for just a little while, the Christian may endure suffering and grief, but we look forward to a future free from sorrow and pain. Despair is not the portion of those who hope in Christ.

Today's Scripture: *"For He has rescued us from the dominion of darkness and has brought us into the kingdom of the Son He loves, in whom we have redemption, the forgiveness of sins" (Colossians 1:13-14).*

Day 7

Praise God in the Heartache

I learned to find solace in praise and worship music. One day I broke open the package of a brand new CD by a Christian rock group. The title song was inspiring, but the selection that brought tears to my eyes was about continuing to honor God with praise when life's circumstances look bleak. The first time I heard this song I hurried to the CD player to turn it off. Too many emotions came rushing to the surface, emotions I worked hard to keep submerged. I realized that I did not want to praise the Lord in the midst of the storm of grief I felt over my mom; rather, I wanted to escape from the heartache altogether! To this end, I found myself avoiding eye contact, emotional intimacy, and meaningful conversation. I performed my duties and fled to the safety of a book, a movie, or to food.

I suppose it is instinctive to draw one's hand away from the hot fire of grief, but I found a divine paradox; if I tried to flee the pain through escapism, I soon found myself overcome by flames of sorrow. "For whoever wants to save his life will lose it," (Mark 8:35).

Grief is like one of those woven finger traps that tighten the harder one pulls. I learned that the only way to escape was to go deeper in, with the Lord at my side and the confidence that He would bring me through. I knew this didn't mean that I should go around with tears in my eyes and a sorrowful countenance. It's just that I needed to stop avoiding the grief issue and to take my sorrows to the Lord's healing balm and comforting arms of solace.

I prayed for the strength to give up avoidance of the Lord, of my mother, and of others God put in my path. As I delved deeper into God's Word and opened my heart to praise, I was delivered from the danger of wasting the discipline of grief.

Today's Scripture: *"For whoever wants to save his life will lose it, but whoever loses his life for me and for the gospel will save it" (Mark 8:35).*

"Be merciful to me, O LORD, for I am in distress; my eyes grow weak with sorrow, my soul and my body with grief ... But I trust in you, O LORD; I say, 'You are my God,' My times are in your hands" (Psalm 31:9, 14-15).

Day 8

The Good Daughter's Dilemma

One evening, Mom was sitting in her chair reading over her day's journal entry. She handed the spiral notebook to me and said, "Look at this. This looks like I'm completely out of it. I don't feel that way now." I took the journal from her and read the following entry:

Monday, October 10: It doesn't seem reasonable not to be upset when I look around me at my nice, pleasant apartment, but do not know really where I am, or why I'm here. Let's see why I'm not—it seems reasonable that at age 81 I must have lost some capability of clear thinking. I know I have one daughter, and that she is living, and a deceased husband. It also seems likely that she would see that her mother was looked after properly. This is what I will assume, and be very grateful to her, and to my Lord God for placing me in these circumstances.

It seems reasonable to proceed as if I know what I am doing—reading, eating, listening to pleasant music. What more could one ask? The book on my lapboard is called Blessings in Disguise, *and it looks as if I have been reading it, so why not proceed?*

My first response to this entry was, oddly enough, anger. I ran to my word processor and typed, "Well, what did I think? Did I believe that I had discovered a cure for Alzheimer's? Did I think that by taking *very good care* of my mother that I could succeed in keeping her from deteriorating? That a handful of vitamins and a walk around the driveway each day would keep this disease from progressing?"

The reason for the fact that I had been struggling to keep patience with my mother was revealed. I had worked hard to keep her from failing, and I had begun to feel a little bit proud of the fruits of my efforts. Whenever she forgot some important detail of living—*yes, Mom, you have a daughter, and yes, she is seeing that you get reasonable care*—I was taking it personally! I felt affronted! How dare she not improve when I'd worked so hard to see that she do so! This kind of thing reflected badly on *me*!

I came to the Lord, and was re-oriented to the truth; my hope was in God alone. I had done my best, but my mother was still failing, and my grief over this fact had expressed itself as anger. I prayed for humility and freedom from pride, and to receive with thanksgiving both the trials and joys God had ordained for me. My hope needed to be in the Lord, and not in myself or in my own efforts. I could not change what was happening to my mother, but I could allow the Lord to change me.

Today's Scripture: *"Let us hold unswervingly to the hope we profess, for He who promised is faithful" (Hebrews 10:23).*

43

Day 9

Bad Feelings and Forgiven Sin

One of the cardinal rules of caring for an Alzheimer patient is that if change needs to occur, it is the caregiver who has to make necessary adjustments. Nevertheless, one day I impatiently asked my mother, for the umpteenth time, to place her lap desk on the left side of her chair rather than the right, because she would knock the trash can over if she pushed it off to the right. Of course, she could not remember my request. I returned to her room a short while later, and there she was; her lap desk lying on the floor to her right, waste basket tumbled over, wadded tissues spilling every which way, and an angelic smile on her face. I didn't say a word, but I'm sure she could tell by my body language, that I was not pleased. I cleaned the mess and came back into my kitchen. I found myself standing in the middle of the floor with clenched fists and tears running down my face. I wasn't angry with Mom; I was sad over her, and I felt rebellious toward the Lord.

I felt an absolute dread of my mother's demise, not just over the fact that she would at some point die; but I was afraid of the loss of function that might happen before that time. The ingredients of the cocktail of grief of which I had unwillingly partaken included terrible pity and love for my mother, anger, resentment, guilt, and fear of the future. This draught was complex and it was bitter. It was as though I didn't want to analyze the components of my pain, but I had no choice about dealing with the results of having drunk such a bitter brew. I didn't feel so good!

The next morning I didn't want to get out of bed. I was aware of my Lord's *still, small, voice* calling me, but I resisted. "It's not you, Lord," I explained. "It's me. I don't want to face the grief and guilt of having treated my mother unfairly."

I finally came to God in prayer. As I opened my mind and heart, the first release and comfort came from remembering that my salvation does not depend on me. If I am faithless, He is faithful (2 Timothy 2:13). If I allow grief, guilt, or pain to cause me to turn away from Him, even then, He will not turn away from me. Next came an awareness of His wonderful compassion for both my mother and for me. He understood, and He had made a way for me to be cleansed of my sinful responses to the burdens He had allowed me to bear. He did not excuse my sin; He forgave it and wiped it away completely!

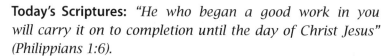

Today's Scriptures: *"He who began a good work in you will carry it on to completion until the day of Christ Jesus" (Philippians 1:6).*

"Continue to work out your salvation with fear and trembling, for it is God who works in you to will and to act according to His good purpose" (Philippians 2:12-13).

Day 10

Obedience

Nothing dulls the perception of God's love and solace as much as lack of obedience. Obedience became even more vital to me when I found myself saying with the Psalmist, "The troubles of my heart have multiplied," (Psalm 25:17).

We Christians tend to forego large sins, but then proceed to disobey the Lord in small ways. In one of C.S. Lewis's *Narnia* tales, *The Voyage of the Dawn Treader,* the young girl, Lucy, is turning the pages of a magical book. She is obedient not to use a powerful spell in order to make herself beautiful, but having been obedient in something so important she quickly disobeys by speaking the words to a lesser spell. Lewis says, "Now Lucy had wanted very badly to try the other spell, the one that made you beautiful beyond the lot of mortals. So she felt that to make up for not having said it, she really would say this one. And all in a hurry, for fear her mind would change, she said the words . . . . "[2] In the midst of the testing time of my mother's Alzheimer's, I obeyed in the big ways. I prayed, sought to act in love, and ministered to my mother's physical needs. But like Lucy, having given up so much that was really important to me; I disobeyed in small ways, medicating my grief by catering to my physical body's desire for comfort. If comfort is one's main goal, then exercise and Godly eating habits become secondary concerns.

I found myself coping with a series of minor health crises as a result of my disobedience. Of much greater concern was the fact that I felt distanced from the Lord. I did not ask, "Why, O LORD, do you stand far off?" (Psalm 10:1). I knew why His voice came to my awareness sounding muffled and far away, as though my head was wrapped in layers of cotton wool. In my heart I knew that by prioritizing my own comfort, I was letting the Lord slip to second place.

Jesus says, "For whoever wants to save his life will lose it, but whoever loses his life for me will find it" (Matthew 16:25). There is a sacrifice involved in obedience; we place at the Savior's feet something that is precious to us, and vow to leave it with Him. It is difficult, but through this small loss there is gain of unfathomable magnitude. We gain intimacy with Christ, oneness with God, and are empowered by the Holy Spirit.

The fruits of obedience are worth the sacrifice and hard work sometimes involved. When we gain a glimpse of our Savior's face, no earthly pleasure can compare.

Today's Scripture: *"Jesus replied, 'If anyone loves me, he will obey my teaching. My Father will love him, and we will come to him and make our home with him. He who does not love me will not obey my teaching. These words you hear are not my own; they belong to the Father who sent me'" (John 14:23-24).*

Chapter Three

Releasing the Bad Stuff

Just when I wanted to exhibit kindness, supportiveness,
and love to my mom, I was suffused by feelings of resentment,
guilt, and anger.

—Linda

Linda was in. Don't complain about how she acts, Anna Ruth.
After all, you raised her.

—Anna Ruth

Day 1

Guilt

*"Let us draw near to God with a sincere heart in full
assurance of faith, having our hearts sprinkled to cleanse
us from a guilty conscience" (Hebrews 10:22).*

*L*ate one evening after Mom had gone to bed, I picked
up her journal and was dismayed to read these words,
"I wonder what percentage of suicides occur because of
boredom?" I felt immediate guilt. Although I was certain
Mother was not truly suicidal; I took her to the doctor. Her
antidepressant medication was judged to be sufficient, and
no change was made.

My real upset came over the fact that, in the moment
she wrote those words, she must have been suffering from
dissatisfaction and boredom. I ran to my word processor
and defensively listed all of the things I did each day for
Mom. It was a lengthy and detailed record that included
provision for conversation, reading materials, music,
exercise, and meals served with a smile. In addition to my
ministrations, my husband served Mom her lunch each day
and would often sit and visit with her during the noon hour.
Even as I added items to my list, I really knew that on busy
days, Mom's emotional and spiritual needs sometimes went

unmet. Despite the extensive record of all my good deeds, I recognized that I carried a constant sense of guilt because I didn't provide adequate happy chatter, entertainment, or social interaction. At this moderate stage of the progression of her disease, I was confident that she was much happier in our home environment than she would have been in any other circumstances we could have provided for her. But the fact remained that I had not been successful in protecting her from that soul withering sense of worthlessness and boredom that can cause such depression for those people we describe as *shut-ins.* Even worse than the sense of failure was the fact that I knew I had no intention of adding to my list of "things to do". I was at capacity, perhaps not of what I was able to do, but of what I was willing to do. And that just caused me to feel more guilt.

I prayed. I received peace and an understanding that I did not have to add *activities director* to my list of responsibilities to Mom. I recognized that the Lord is my mother's provider, and that I am not the only person through whom He works to bless her days. The Lord gently brought to my remembrance the many gestures of kindness and love that came to Mom from concerned friends and loved ones. I was able to release the self-condemnation and defensiveness I'd felt, and to rest in the assurance of God's compassion and provision for both my mother and for me.

Today's Scripture: *"This then is how we know that we belong to the truth, and how we set our hearts at rest in His presence whenever our hearts condemn us. For God is greater than our hearts, and He knows everything" (1 John 3:19-20).*

Caregiving Strategy

If symptoms of depression occur, your loved one must see a physician for an accurate diagnosis. Not only is depression a common accompaniment to dementia, it can actually mimic Alzheimer's disease or other forms of dementia. A professional evaluation is necessary.

Day 2

Resentment

"The godless in heart harbor resentment" (Job 36:13).

$\mathcal{A}$ cold that threatened me for a solid week finally conquered my efforts to thwart it. I battled valiantly with green tea, zinc supplements, and prayer; but the virus continued its advance, marking territory gained with flags of raging sore throat and congested sinuses.

Late on a Sunday evening I was nursing a fairly severe case of self-pity and was in the kitchen heating a kettle for a cup of herbal tea before bedtime. As I waited for the kettle to boil, I morosely examined the labels on two bottles of pills, weighing the advantages of acetaminophen versus ibuprofen for sore throat pain. There came a cry from Mother's room closely followed by John's urgent summons for me to come quickly.

Mother had tripped on the edge of the braided rug and had fallen hard onto her left side. She clutched her shoulder and moaned with pain, and when we attempted to lift her she cried out. We are blessed to have two emergency medical technicians in our family circle, and we called them for advice. They came immediately. With expertise and strength, they eased Mom into a standing position, and five hours of adventure ensued as we made a trip to the emergency room. We were greeted at the door by a bleary eyed nurse who confided that she was on her fourth twelve hour shift in a week, and was worn out. She consulted an equally weary looking colleague, and together they poked, prodded, x-rayed, and finally trussed Mother's arm into a sling. They then sent her back home with us. The instructions were as follows: "No surgery required, see an orthopedist in a week, keep the arm immobilized." The nurse brightened considerably as we made preparations to depart. It was a slow night in the ER and I had the distinct feeling that if we had not interrupted that she would have been able to catch up with her other duties; perhaps she had a backlog of paperwork waiting. She cheerily waved goodbye as we pulled out of the hospital parking lot. She was happy to see us go. I confess that I would have been equally happy to have left my mother at the hospital. A little voice in my head was saying, "You don't feel well. You ought not to have to exert yourself like this at 2:30 AM."

After Mom's accident I struggled with resentment. She was like a child who did not question a parent's ministrations, and even took them as her due. But I was a former child and my mother had given up all pretense of ministering to me. The person who was supposed to be my caregiver required caregiving from me, even though I was sick. The thoughts that fueled my bad feelings did not stand up under the Lord's light. After our return from the hospital I found myself failing to greet Mother with kind and supportive words when she called for me in the night. I regressed to one syllable grunts as I shuffled resentfully to her side. Fortunately, she remained annoyingly oblivious to my pathetic coughing and groaning, as well as to my judgmental desire to punish her for all the ways she had failed me. I had to turn to the Lord as my caregiver, and stop resenting my mother for not taking care of me.

Today's Scriptures: *"The LORD is with me; He is my helper" (Psalm 118:7).*

"Even if my father and mother abandon me, the Lord will hold me close" (Psalm 27:10, NLT).

Day 3

If Only I Was Perfect

*M*other's broken shoulder was a blessing in disguise. Up to that point she had needed my help with bathing but had resisted my offers of aid. Now as she struggled with the painful shoulder, she recognized that she had to have help. Understandably though, some angst remained. She was embarrassed and in pain, and my bumbling efforts to be of assistance were exasperating for her. For my part, I had difficulty responding with kindness to her obvious resentment of me. One particularly memorable verbal exchange ended with Mother throwing a wet washcloth in my general direction. It missed, but I was offended just the same. That evening I made the following tongue-in-cheek entry in my journal:

> *Unfortunately, neither my mother nor I are sin-free. If we were both saintly in our words and actions toward one another, life would be so easy. Even if just one of us was perfect, our relationship could thrive. I try so hard to be perfect. I succeed beautifully until the moment when my mother is not perfect toward me.*

My Scripture reading for the day included a passage from Deuteronomy 7, which states that the Israelites were to purge the Promised Land of its evil inhabitants little by little. I found this encouraging because I realized that even if I was not yet perfect; I did have God's promise that I was in the process of being perfected *little by little.*

Sometimes a cleansing and purging can happen instantaneously, but more often we are healed little by little of the sins that separate us from God. This happens as we walk forward in Him, seeking His face through Scripture and prayer.

There is always a struggle to take accountability for my sinfulness before the Lord. Some of my sins come to me only by association and aren't really mine. These release their hold easily; sometimes I really don't know that something is wrong until the Lord tells me. Some sins I acquired through, or in response to environmental influences. These are tougher because I want to cast blame and indulge in resentment against anyone who caused me harm. And, many of my sins are mine alone, due entirely to my unique inclination toward sin.

The Lord does not differentiate between sins. It's as though I purchased the same product from several different stores and the Lord doesn't make a distinction as to where I shopped for my particular brand.

Every variety of sin leaves the same sort of stain on our souls, and Jesus is the cleansing agent for it all.

Today's Scriptures: *"The LORD will drive out those nations before you, little by little" (Deuteronomy 7:22).*

"On that day a fountain will be opened to the house of David and the inhabitants of Jerusalem, to cleanse them from sin and impurity" (Zechariah 13:1).

"Christ loved the church and gave himself up for her to make her holy, cleansing her by the washing with water through the word, and to present her to himself as a radiant church, without stain or wrinkle or any other blemish, but holy and blameless" (Ephesians 5:25b-27).

Day 4

Disturber of Mom's Peace

At church one Sunday morning, a former Christian Youth Fellowship student of my mother's asked me how she was doing. I described how she liked to sit in her recliner reading a book. I told him that she enjoyed soft music playing in the background, and that she often spoke of feeling at peace.

He raised an eyebrow and said, "Doesn't sound so bad."

As I walked to my car I realized that the resentment I felt toward Mom centered on this very thought; she really did seem to have it pretty good. While I struggled with fear over finances, and cringed beneath the hand that was upraised to deal me the blows of her inevitable decline and death; she was not in the least worried about the future. She was unconcerned. She had no physical aches or pains other than a knee that gave a twinge on our short walks. She had no worries at all about food, clothing, or money. She had a childlike confidence and expectation that all of these things were being handled for her. She liked her chair, her food, her music, her books, and her cat. She coped with the things she did not like by utilizing a kind of emotional and mental detachment, which I was not convinced was conducive toward helping her to maintain cognitive function. I had been irritated by this, but maybe it was just a normal end of life withdrawing from the things of this world.

I was hurting from grief and from fear of the approaching pain of separation from my mother. It was not fair of me to resent her because she was not in pain too. If my mother's life was a still and peaceful pool of water, I was too often the stone that disturbed the clear surface of her confidence and peace. I bustled around as though I had the cares of the world on my shoulders, when in reality the Lord was providing for me just as surely as He had provided for her. One of my mother's journal entries spoke about her own mother's death. She said:

> I can remember the years when I felt the earth would stop turning without my mother on it. Of course, life does go on, but not with the same joy, and when I'm gone life will go right on too, thank you, Lord.

When I read these words I recognized that I, like my mother before me, was grieved to be faced with loss of the joy of having a mother.

I prayed that the Lord would prevent me from poisoning the remaining time I had with Mom with anger toward her because she was leaving me. Only in the Lord could I do the work required of me as a caregiver, be an emotional support to my mother, and manage to keep my equilibrium. I released fear, and prayed not to be a disturbance of the peace God had ordained for my mother.

Today's Scripture: *"The LORD is gracious and righteous; our God is full of compassion. The LORD protects the simple-hearted; when I was in great need, He saved me. Be at rest once more, O my soul, for the LORD has been good to you"* *(Psalm 116:5-7).*

Day 5

Dark Thoughts

Those who know me best are well aware that I did not walk meekly through the trials associated with my mother's illness. I cried, sometimes loudly. I was irritable. I kept my mouth shut while performing caregiving duties, and then vented my feelings at my husband in order to release the pressure of frustrating interchanges with Mother. I suffered all of the negative emotions of anger, resentment, fear, and doubt; and about the only thing I did right was to continue to cry out to the Lord.

Thus, I generally came through in fairly good shape, strengthened by Scripture, by friends who prayed for me, and by God's grace. But there were more difficult days as well, days when my physical endurance had reached its limits, when caregiving duties conflicted with my other roles as wife and mother; times when I came to the end of my own strength and failed to appropriate the Lord's help.

It was on a day such as this that I recorded the following journal entry:

I have just filled two pages with words that would cause just about anyone to cringe. I used descriptors such as hate *and* resent, *and gave vent to the buried and secret desire that people who have hurt me would vanish from the face of the planet. My anger was not reserved for my mother. No one I love was safe from my tirade of words.*

I described in detail the cleaning up of spilled coffee and yellow stained bed linens. I described piles of dirty laundry with a vividness that should be reserved for annotating those things that are beautiful and praiseworthy. I passed judgment with a vengeance and then, of course, fell into self-judgment, which is one of the most painful results of casting blame.

I'm done, now, Lord. Forgive me. I forgive those I named in my lengthy list of wrongs. I forgive because you have forgiven me. I know that you have provided for me.

Well, praise the Lord for an afternoon of solitude, for the fact that I unleashed my word processor and not my tongue, and most especially for the delete key on my computer keyboard! I will wipe away those angry words and think of the way your blood has wiped away my sins, Lord.

Thank You.

Caregiving was not the tidy and organized venture I would have chosen, but God strengthened me. I learned that it is better to be strengthened to bear a load than it is to escape from the burden altogether. Partaking of God's strength is much to be preferred over cowering in my own weakness. I found His grace to be sufficient for my every need.

Today's Scripture: *"Though I sit in darkness, the LORD will be my light" (Micah 7:8b).*

Insight: If you are a person who is disturbed by disorganization, you will need special prayer as you step into the role of caregiver. Pray to be gifted with hunger for Scripture and be sure to spend much time at Jesus' feet. The beauty of the perfection of His presence satisfies the heart's need for order.

Day 6

Judge Not!

I was repeatedly reminded of the necessity of keeping my heart clean of resentment. When I first became Mom's caregiver I harbored anger toward her because she no longer felt an inclination to *do* for me. I found that every drop of resentment I'd held toward her over the years surfaced, and my behavior was quite childish. "Yeah, you won't (can't?) make your own coffee and you expect me to do it for you ... and then there was that time 34 years ago when ..."

Resentment is a form of passing judgment on another person, and the Bible says quite clearly, *don't do it*. When I harbored resentment toward my mother, I became defensive in my relationship with my daughter because I expected her to judge me in the same way I had judged my mother. And so, manipulated by my own sin, I took extraordinary measures to avoid being judged as I had judged.

It's ironic that I was able to simultaneously insist upon doing that which I did not want to do, while also resenting the self-imposed feeling that I had to do it. An example of this silliness is the story of our family's Sunday gatherings. My mother had always invited all of us to her home for Sunday dinner. It was a relaxing time (for everyone but Mother) and I didn't realize how much I'd looked forward to those weekly respites until they stopped. Before I knew that my mom was sick (and to be honest, for quite some time after) I was very upset with her for no longer inviting us to eat at her table. Oh how I missed the weekly gatherings, and how I resented my mother for no longer ministering to me in this way. I judged her for her failure to meet my needs.

A few months later, I found myself to be the new designated cook for Sunday gatherings. Still reeling from my mother's diagnosis, but determined not to be judged as I had judged, I continued to insist that every family member flock to my home for a meal each week. I was tired, I was grieving, and I did not want to be planning and cooking huge meals each week, but I did it anyway. I was afraid my children would judge me as I had judged my own mother.

Judging others doubles back and causes the one passing the judgment to be bound by his or her own sin. "Judge not that ye be not judged," says God's Word. Under the sentence of our own judgment of others, we fall into the bondage of having to reap what we have sown.

Today's Scripture: *"Do not judge, and you will not be judged. Do not condemn, and you will not be condemned. Forgive, and you will be forgiven" (Luke 6:37).*

Day 7

Love Them With God's Love

Years ago I had the privilege of mentoring a bright and talented young woman who had been assigned to me as a student teacher. I prayed for her, provided her with teaching resources, and all in all felt somewhat self-congratulatory about the fine example I was setting for her. But one day, with the guilelessness of youth she said, "You know, I just love the kindergarten teacher. She is just so kind and sweet all of the time. And she isn't the least bit ...," here she struggled for words, cast a sidelong glance at me and then quickly averted her eyes and completed her sentence, "flippant."

Flippant? I was stung. My student teacher had clearly revealed to me that, unlike the perfect kindergarten teacher, I had been judged to be flippant! Worse yet, I recognized that her assessment of me was correct. I loved to make people laugh and had developed a sarcastic, superficial manner of bantering about my job and my life. I had fallen into the habit of looking for humor in every situation, and when the foibles of my fellow human beings took the brunt of my running commentary, my foolish talk strayed into the territory of sin.

In the years that followed this revelation, I liked to think that I had made progress in controlling my tongue, but

68

under the stress of feeling judged or mistreated I definitely regressed. During one difficult stretch of time when I had sustained some particularly painful blows to my heart, I indulged in negative thoughts toward the people I perceived to be responsible for my pain. In a conversation with a friend I said in a joking manner, "Oh, you think you're bad? I have been wishing that those individuals who have caused me hurt would just disappear from the face of the earth so that I wouldn't have to bother with them anymore!"

The Lord was not amused by either this comment or the sin behind it. In prayer I repented of these words that spoke in a joking way about lives the Lord holds precious. As I prayed this thought came, "When I meet darkness, it can't invade where there is light. Like is drawn to like. Most times the outrage I feel at the shortcomings of other people occurs because there is a kindred darkness in me."

Once again I prayed, "Lord forgive me for passing judgment on others and forgive my sinful words. Let me forgive them as you have forgiven me, and love them with your love."

Today's Scripture: *"Anyone who claims to be in the light but hates his brother is still in the darkness. Whoever loves his brother lives in the light, and there is nothing in him to make him stumble. But whoever hates his brother is in the darkness and walks around in the darkness; he does not know where he is going because the darkness has blinded him" (1 John 2:8-11).*

Day 8

I'll Never Catch Up

I learned that apart from a constant realignment with the Lord, my human heart fell toward resentment and rebellion just as the needle on a compass swings north.

Caregiving required a love and a patience that I did not possess apart from the Lord. God did not give me any leeway at all for being short tempered with my mother. Every devotion time left me with the clear mandate to love as I had been loved by God, and to forgive as I'd been forgiven.

One evening I was preparing a meal for my mother, and my thoughts were not charitable. It's amazing how illogical I could be in my resentment! I felt absolutely righteous as I resented my poor mother because she was no longer able to care for herself, much less take care of my needs. However, I remembered to pray and there came the thought, "How many meals has your mother prepared for you?"

I found a calculator and came up with a very conservative estimate. Three meals a day to age five (not counting the middle of the night feedings an infant requires) and then two meals a day to age 18 totaled 14,965. Because my mother prepared family dinners each Sunday evening, and my husband, children, and I lived close enough to partake, she continued to feed me once a week for the next 32 years. I pressed more buttons on the calculator and discovered that over my lifetime, my mother had prepared approximately 17,000 meals for me. A little more math revealed that even if I were to prepare three meals a day for Mom for the rest of her life I would still fall far short of the number of breakfasts, lunches and dinners my mother had set before me.

Humbled, I acknowledged the fact that there was not one service I carried out for my mother that she had not performed hundreds of times more for me. I could never catch up.

As I pondered the contrast of my mother's years of sacrifice of time and love for me with my small gifts of service to her, I thought of the enormity of God's sacrifice in His gift of Jesus Christ. In light of God's great love, the small sacrifices He asked of me as I ministered to my mother were not only His due, but a joy and a privilege to offer.

Today's Scripture: *"Whatever you do, work at it with all your heart, as working for the Lord, not for men, since you know that you will receive an inheritance from the Lord as a reward. It is the Lord Christ you are serving"* (Colossians 3:23-24).

Caregiving Strategy

Make a list of the ways you have been blessed through the life of your loved one, asking for the Lord's help to bring these things to mind. This is a bittersweet exercise, but valuable both in helping you to express gratitude to your dementia patient, and as a reminder that before you were the caregiver, you were the recipient of much care. If the

71

person who is receiving your care was harmful to you in the past, this task becomes more difficult, but not impossible. The Lord will bring to your mind ways in which this person's life has blessed your life and those of others—even if the blessing came as a result of the strengths you gained by doing without his or her support.

Day 9

Repentance

*A*s I became an unwilling observer of my mother's slow decline I was subject to a host of unwanted memories and emotions. I found myself fuming not only over real or imagined injuries that I had received from my mother; I was angry with everyone! At the precise time when I wanted to be loving, compassionate, and kind toward my mother and husband I found myself to be short-tempered and rude. I was ashamed of myself and prayed for a spirit of repentance. How carefully I had stored up anger and bitterness against my *beloved enemies*, those closest to me who had inevitably hurt my heart as we traveled along together.

One of my journal entries from that time of anger says:

I can see quite clearly the wrongs in one who has hurt me, but apart from God's grace I am unable to look at my own sinful heart. The misconception that keeps me from being able to admit wrong is that if I am wrong, then those who hurt me must be right. This is a heart-crushing idea that negates all the suffering I've endured at the hands of other people, and I can't accept it. However, if I can acknowledge that all of my circumstances are engineered by the Lord and are used to sculpt and form me according to His will; I have taken the first step toward acceptance of the painful sections of the path I've traveled. The other part of this understanding is the realization that my confession of sin does not negate the sin of the other party. God hears my cries of pain and I can trust Him to take action on my behalf.

What I cannot expect is to participate in the judgment or retribution that God brings down on the heads of those who have caused me pain. Vengeance belongs to the Lord. Any sense of entitlement I feel as a result of having suffered wrong at the hands of another human being will lead me to sin. Apart from the Lord, the pain of being a victim of injustice plows my heart with hurt, making it a fertile ground for the growth of vindictive anger, fear that I won't receive what is rightfully mine, and a desire of retribution. I administer judgment in the form of a critical spirit, harsh words, withdrawal from emotional connectedness, and a cold heart toward the suffering of others.

The balancing of the scales of justice is entirely in God's hands. I sin when I harbor a desire to show them all. *Revelation 3:9 says that the Lord will make all those who are of the "synagogue of Satan" fall down at my feet and acknowledge that God has loved me, but I want them to fall down at my feet and acknowledge that I was right and they were wrong. And I don't mind viewing anybody who has hurt me as being a member of the synagogue of Satan! Again I trespass on ground that belongs exclusively to God; He is the only one qualified to judge.*

It is humbling to finally arrive at the realization that the Lord's love is so vast that He loves and freely forgives a prodigal. The elder brother was a proud and bitter man who could not forgive his brother as the father had forgiven. "Lord, please cleanse me of pride and forgive me for resentment and bitterness against those you have loved."

When I am unable to forgive, I risk a judgment day when I will have to fall down at the feet of those I viewed as perpetrators of wrongdoing toward me, and acknowledge that God has loved them. All things come to me from God's hand and His alone, and vengeance belongs solely to Him.

I prayed for the ability to love as I had been loved, to forgive as I had been forgiven, and for cleansing from bitterness in order to make way for the fruit of the Holy Spirit to be manifested in my life. The recognition that I had suffered so little compared to the Lord's suffering on my behalf led me to pray to be transformed into a closer approximation of His likeness, so that I could develop holy habits of manifesting God's love and acceptance to others.

Today's Scripture: *"When they hurled their insults at Him, He did not retaliate; when He suffered, He made no threats. Instead, He entrusted himself to Him who judges justly. He himself bore our sins in His body on the tree so that we might die to sins and live for righteousness; by His wounds you have been healed. For you were like sheep going astray, but now you have returned to the Shepherd and Overseer of your souls" (1 Peter 2:23-25).*

Day 10

Let Me Do That for You

Sometimes the Lord speaks to me just at the moment when I begin to awaken, before my mind becomes busy with my ever present list of things to do. In order to capture those thoughts that come in the predawn stillness, I've learned to keep a notepad and a pen on my bedside table. One morning I awoke to find that in the night I had scribbled these words: "You can't say, 'Let me do that for you,' to your mother if you are still angry that she is not *doing* for you."

I had already learned that my mother was relieved whenever I could say, "Don't you worry about this. I will take care of it for you." I knew that one of the most difficult aspects of Alzheimer's for the person with the disease is the confusion that results from not understanding one's environment. The plaques and tangles that are characteristic of the Alzheimer's diseased brain caused Mom to begin to have difficulty speaking and understanding speech, and this resulted in disorientation and confusion. Mom badly needed someone she trusted to reassure her and to provide her the comfort of knowing that all of her responsibilities were being handled for her. However, this *in the head* knowledge had not reached my heart.

I had responded to my mother's need for me to take care of her out of the emotional deficit I felt from no longer having a mother to lean on, rather than out of the knowledge

I had gained about the disease that had attacked her brain. My response to Mom's need of me had been resentful as opposed to gracious. Caught up in grief over the loss of being the recipient of motherly care, I was not yet ready to reverse roles and become the supplier of my mother's needs. I felt like the Israelites in Exodus 5. They were told to make more bricks, while the straw necessary to the brick making process was withheld. Serving my mother out of the deficit I felt in my heart was hard labor.

I recognized that the place in my heart that had once been filled with my mother's nurture and care now needed to be filled with the Lord. A Scripture memorized long ago, Isaiah 6:1, came to mind as I remembered that Isaiah saw the Lord in the year that his king died. In *My Utmost for His Highest*, Oswald Chambers refers to this revelation given to Isaiah and says, "Our soul's personal history with God is often an account of the death of our heroes. Over and over again God has to remove our friends to put himself in their place, and that is when we falter, fail, and become discouraged. Let me think about this personally—when the person died who represented for me all that God was, did I give up on everything in life? Did I become ill or disheartened? Or did I do as Isaiah did and see the Lord?"[3]

Today's Scripture: *"In the year that King Uzziah died, I saw the Lord seated on a throne, high and exalted, and the train of His robe filled the temple" (Isaiah 6:1).*

Caregiver's Prayer

Father, forgive my anger over the deficit in my heart. Please fill my emptiness with your Spirit. Open my eyes to see new manifestations of your power, presence and provision for my life. And grant me grace to say in love, *let me do that for you.* Amen.

Chapter Four

Honor and Respect

My mother had been a girl whose favorite class in school was
journalism, a young woman on her own in Kansas City,
a bride who raised a garden and canned her own vegetables,
and a mother. She had taught Sunday school, cooked for
countless church suppers, and had been a Christian Youth
Fellowship leader for junior high youth in her community.
I had to make a conscious effort to look beyond the facade of
old age and fading memory in order to honor her not only as
my parent, but also as the accomplished and richly experienced
individual that she was.

—Linda

When I feel an occasional tug of loneliness
I remember how good the Lord has been all these years,
and I know that He is still with me.

—Anna Ruth

Day 1

Trading Tears for Smiles

*W*hen I was a child, I was loved unconditionally by my mother. Even when I frightened or exasperated her, I was confident that she would eventually enfold me in the safe haven of her arms and forgive me. I remember that I once hid from her under a bush on the lawn of our little farm house. I felt secure and delightfully disguised as I peered out through the greenery, and at age three the sight of my mother pacing back and forth across the lawn shouting my name in tones of rising panic gave me a sense of infantile power. Although the poor woman was nearing hysteria when I finally strolled out, I was not in the least concerned. She clung to me, covered me with kisses, and I probably got a cookie out of the deal. When I became a parent myself I possessed a similar extravagance of love toward my own children. My little ones moved about in their carefully protected world with freedom and the confidence that came from the fact that they knew Mommy thought they were wonderful. As a caregiver, I so wanted to be able to bless my mother with a similar environment of love and acceptance.

For a time, it was a daily struggle. Anger muddied the clear waters of love and kept us from communicating acceptance and love to one another. Past hurts and present grief all too often led me to sinful responses toward Mom that were rarely based on her behaviors in the present. In other words, she didn't deserve it. And even if she was wrong, I remained accountable to the Lord for my responses to her.

The first stanza of the great hymn "What a Friend We Have in Jesus" perfectly expresses how we deprive ourselves of peace when we fail to bring everything to the Lord, "Oh what peace we often forfeit, oh what needless pain we bear, all because we do not carry everything to God in prayer."[4] I confessed my resentful behaviors toward Mom to the members of my Bible study, and during prayer time I asked God's forgiveness. To my discomfort, I found that grief came bubbling up when resentment departed. I recognized that I had preferred the cold detachment of resentment to the scalding helplessness of grief. But of course, I had been carrying both burdens and had been using anger and resentment as a sort of hardened shell in an attempt to protect myself from having to experience the underlying grief. The Lord wanted me to release my sins and sorrows to Him, not to repress them and thus allow them to taint my words and actions.

I read an old Jewish saying awhile back that said, "When a father helps a son, both smile; but when a son must help his father, both weep." This is the tragedy of Alzheimer's, but in casting my cares on the Lord I found a way to smile again with Mom.

Today's Scripture: *"Cast all your anxiety on Him, because He cares for you" (1 Peter 5:7).*

Insight: There is no other interaction with my mother that is so satisfying as laughing together. Our cat provides many opportunities for shared laughter. I challenge you to find a way to laugh with your loved one. Pray for the Lord's guidance, and He will help you to smile together again.

Day 2

Love Is Not Easily Offended

I often say that Alzheimer patients have trouble *connecting the dots*. It took some time for me to recognize that Mom did not make connections between the comforts that surrounded her and my labor on her behalf. She often expressed thanksgiving to God, but she no longer seemed to know how much I craved her praise and her gratitude, and I was offended by this.

My husband, John, didn't do much actual caregiving of Mom, but would often stop by just to visit with her. By contrast, when I came to her room I didn't always take time for the finer points of social niceties. I would hand her medications to swallow, inform her that it was time for a shower, or get her up to exercise.

One night John and I were talking just outside Mom's room. John's voice is deep, and carried through the door. When I opened Mom's door and walked through she looked up, her face alight, expecting to see John. When she saw that it was me, her face fell. I was *deeply* offended! I brought my complaints before the Lord and as I prayed I wrote the following words:

> *Do not childishly crave your mother's expressions of approval or demand that she recognize all you are*

going through. God knows. Allow her the dignity of feeling that she is paying her way. Find ways to assure her that she is a blessing and an asset to you rather than a burden. Tell her often how glad you are that she is in your home. God is with you. If you act burdened and communicate your stress to your mother, you are in sin against the Lord, who has provided for you.

Show gratitude to her. All she has is being transferred into your hands. Do not act as though this is your due because you are caring for her. Don't be arrogant. If she didn't have a penny you would still owe her a great debt not only for her years of love and sacrifice for you, but because it was through her that you received the gift of life, and you are to honor her. Above that debt is your debt to Jesus Christ and your obligation to love and to care for those He loves.

Spend time in fellowship with her. Take time to talk with her and to laugh with her. She is not just your charge or your responsibility, she is your mother. Enjoy her. Pray for her. Do not distance yourself from her in an effort to avoid the sorrow of empathy for her. This hardens your heart to her emotions.

I recognized that I needed to worry less about whether I was treated fairly, and more about whether I was manifesting God's love to those around me.

Today's Scripture: *"If we claim to have fellowship with Him yet walk in the darkness, we lie and do not live by the truth. But if we walk in the light as He is in the light, we have fellowship with one another, and the blood of Jesus, His Son, purifies us from all sin" (1 John 1:6-8).*

Day 3

What Not to Do

One evening I went to bed feeling exhausted, but I could not sleep. I stared at the ceiling, pondering the various ways I'd botched my caregiving duties for the day. I finally sat up and pulled a spiral notebook from my bedside table, turned to a crisp new page and across the top wrote in bold letters, *The Alzheimer's Caregiver's Guide of What NOT to Do or Say.* I began this literary treasure with a list of words best not spoken to one's ailing and frail parent; gems of wisdom gleaned from saying the wrong (a.k.a. sinful) thing and then carefully observing the consequences. Here, in part, is that list:

1. When an Alzheimer patient says, "I forgot," the kind and supportive caregiver does not reply, "No joking."

2. When an elderly parent spills her orange juice and doesn't clean it up and it is found three hours later after it's been tracked all over the floor, the loving and prayerful caregiver does not say, "Do you just stay up nights thinking of ways to make my job harder?"

3. When an Alzheimer patient tells the Christmas tree how pretty it is the compassionate caregiver does not make a comment such as the following: "Mother, when you talk to inanimate objects you sound crazy as a loon."

But for the fact that this particular Alzheimer patient was quite well equipped with the skills needed to handle her errant daughter, the words listed above would have been a clear-cut case for the Alzheimer Care Police to be dispatched in order to rescue my mother and to charge me with cruelty to the elderly. However, Mom was not defenseless.

On the day in question I'd had *One of Those Days.* It was late, and I'd thought Mom to be tucked safely in bed, when she appeared at the doorway and said, "I feel confused." I comforted her, tucked her back in, and said a prayer with her. I came back out and sat down.

Mom appeared again. "I don't seem to have any washcloths," she said. I provided the washcloths, waited until she was back in bed, sat with her a bit, and talked to her. I shut the door to her apartment only to hear it open again five minutes later. "Do you ever have times when you don't know who you are or why you are here?" she asked.

I was done with kindness for the day and said, "Nope. I always know who I am."

She gave me an exasperated look and in a snappy and 100% the mother-I've-always-known-voice she replied, "Well, goody for you!" She turned on her heel and returned to her room.

A few minutes later I slunk to her door and opened it timidly. Her eyes were still sparking dangerously and I inquired politely and with as much compassion as I could muster, "Mama, do you know your name? Is that what is wrong?"

She said, "Yes, Linda, I know my name, that is not what I meant." Her Bible was open in her lap and she ignored me and began to read from the Word. And so I left her with the only *one* who could meet the needs of her heart, but sleeplessness was my penalty for my sins of the tongue. I asked God's forgiveness; and once again Mom and I were covered by grace even when my behavior was textbook *What Not to Do!*

Today's Scripture: *"The LORD will perfect that which concerneth me: thy mercy, O LORD, endureth for ever: forsake not the works of thine own hands" (Psalm 138:8 KJV).*

Day 4

The White Eagle Tavern

*E*ach evening after I helped Mom into bed, I pulled the rocking chair into her room and sat by her bedside. It was a peaceful time, and a time for visiting together unencumbered by our roles of caregiver and patient. Just a question or two would elicit a flow of memories, and nearly every evening I learned something new about my mother's past or family history.

One Saturday night in April, our son Jonathan attended his junior/senior prom. I told Mother about the festivities surrounding his special night. Jon and his date were to arrive at the prom in unique style, riding in a wagon drawn by draft horses. When Mom heard this she laughed softly and related the following story:

"When I was a junior in high school, both my best friend and I were dating sophomores. Sophomores weren't allowed to attend the prom, so Norma Ruth and I went together. We had fun, but when it was time to go home we were still in high spirits and didn't feel that the evening should be over just yet. So, we were very daring. We walked right down the middle of Main Street, straight out to the White Eagle Tavern where we boldly walked right in, sat down, and ordered cokes." She laughed again, "Our boyfriends were just furious when they found out what we had done."

I laughed incredulously but inside I felt a little shocked. "What about your parents?" I asked.

"Oh," she said breezily, "When I was in high school I stayed in town during the week because it was so far out to the home place. The older couple I stayed with just left the front door open and I could come home whenever I wanted!"

Throughout the years my perception of my mother transitioned from viewing her as the one who met my needs to a role reversal as I became her caregiver. Was there ever a time when I viewed her as an individual apart from my need of her or hers of me? The Lord knew my mother from before her birth and could see the whole of her life and personality, from the beginning of her life to the end. By contrast I had known only the portion of my mother's character and life labeled "Linda's mother." My perspective of her life was being expanded. In my imagination I could now see her not only as my mother, but also as a daring 16-year-old girl clad in a prom dress, sipping sodas with her best friend in the White Eagle Tavern at 3:00 AM.

Today's Scripture: *"For you created my inmost being; you knit me together in my mother's womb ... All the days ordained for me were written in your book before one of them came to be" (Psalm 139:13,16).*

Caregiving Strategy

Behind the dementia patient's facade of age and disease is an individual who is a composite of a rich history woven of unique life experiences. If available, old photo albums are wonderful catalysts for memories. As you listen to the stories elicited by the photos there is the opportunity to validate and honor your loved one's history.

Day 5

Learning to Empathize With Mom

*M*om had lived with us a year when I broke a bone in my foot and had to wear a non-weight-bearing cast. This temporary handicap was an exercise in endurance. Hauling myself around on crutches strained muscles that I had probably not used since I had swung from the parallel bars on the playground of Crestview Elementary School. I used to hike myself up, legs dangling and arms stiff; and then *walk* the length of the bars with my entire body weight supported by my hands and arms. Approximately forty years had passed since such gymnastics were enjoyable or even possible for me.

As I hobbled from task to task dragging my cast behind me and bemoaning my aching muscles, a rueful knowledge began to dawn: God was making a point. I had the distinct impression that He had allowed me a temporary handicap in order to give me a taste of what it was like to be elderly. The all over muscle aches I experienced from using the crutches mimicked the arthritis my mother felt in her joints. Once I sat down I really didn't want to stand up again. I was content to sit in a chair with my foot propped comfortably, and I was all too willing to avoid the discomfort of getting out of bed in the morning. I had felt impatient with my mother when she exhibited these same behaviors.

The word, "lazy," had come to mind when Mom protested going on our short nightly walks. It would have indeed been lazy to have protested embarking on a quarter mile walk from my usual perspective of health and vitality. But if one's physical handicap made that walk feel like a five mile hike, well, then, we must reconsider. No one likes pain. If I had been required to walk a quarter mile on those crutches I would *really* have complained.

I was learning humility. At the beginning of my ordeal I had found myself balancing on one foot and clutching my brand new crutches while my husband and a male store clerk surveyed me from behind and discussed which size wheelchair I might need. I was unable to negotiate a turn on the crutches in order to glare at them both. At least they didn't pull out a measuring tape. Haughtily (and with a good deal of wishful thinking) I said, "I'll take a size 'small', please."

How often had I robbed my mother of dignity by discussing some detail of her personal information with my husband or daughter within her hearing?

As I attempted to learn to use crutches I made lots of mistakes. Tasks that were simple when I stood on my own two feet became impossibly complicated when negotiated while balanced on one foot and two crutches. I nearly fell several times, and once, when a can of soda spilled, I unthinkingly grabbed for it and ended up lying on the floor in a puddle of diet cola. When my mother broke her shoulder in a similar mishap, I am afraid my attitude was that she should have been more careful.

I saw the world from a completely different perspective as I wheeled around the kitchen in an office chair propelled by my one good foot. I was inefficient. Although I'm the one who planned my kitchen and stocked the pantry and shelves, it was as though my brain had to be rewired. Nothing was automatic now. For example, in order to reach the spice cupboard I had to roll to the cabinet, carefully stand, and reach high while balanced on one foot. This was a whole new set of skills for my brain's file on how to assemble the ingredients for a casserole. The Lord was showing me how difficult it was for my mother to negotiate once familiar tasks while dealing with the handicap of brain cells that were no longer firing properly.

I wore the cast for three weeks and prayed that this brief time was adequate to enable me to learn compassion for my mother.

Today's Scripture: *"Finally, all of you, live in harmony with one another; be sympathetic, love as brothers, be compassionate and humble" (1 Peter 3:8).*

Day 6

Hurt Pride

*A*s a caregiver, I attempted to gain knowledge that would help me to find ways to make life easier for both Mom and myself. I attended several meetings of the local chapter of the Alzheimer's Association, I subscribed to newsletters about elder care, and I did internet research. I even remembered to pray for wisdom, but I neglected one important point. I had a problem with pride, and wisdom will not dwell alongside a prideful spirit. Wisdom hates pride and arrogance. (See Proverbs 8:12-13.)

So many people told me what a lovely thing I had done for my mother by taking her into my home that I began to feel I had done something unusually generous and worthy of praise. I felt a little bit noble, and this fed my pride. The fact was that each step of the way God had provided for us richly, orchestrating circumstances in ways that I could not possibly have conceived, much less brought into reality. I was taking credit unto myself for work that God had done, and this is dangerous. We serve a gracious and merciful God, but His patience can be tested. I remembered the Israelites' punishment when God finally became angry with their rebellion against Him. Moses reminded them that in the desert they had seen how the Lord had provided for them, and yet, "In spite of this, you did not trust the LORD your

God, who went ahead of you on your journey," (Deuteronomy 1:31-33). Those people who failed to recognize that all their blessings were from the Lord were not allowed to enter the Promised Land (See Deuteronomy 1:35.)

Pride is always an ugly sin, but it is particularly reprehensible in someone who carries responsibility for a weaker or childlike person. Pride must always be right, and pride cannot receive an offense. In my interactions with my mother I found that I could correctly analyze what portion of my reaction to any slight was due to hurt pride by measuring the degree of anger I felt. When pride is humiliated, rage results. Legitimate hurt can be healed; pride must be purged.

Today's Scripture: *"God opposes the proud but gives grace to the humble" (James 4:6).*

Day 7

Lighting Is Important

One dark winter afternoon I had a few minutes to myself. I settled into an old overstuffed chair, drew a blanket around me against the chill, and picked up a home decorating magazine. As I flipped through the pages I happened onto an article about lighting. It was interesting and contained information about how mood and energy levels can be affected by the type and amount of light in a room.

A few days later I had the opportunity to observe this phenomenon firsthand. My daughter and I were shopping and, as I'm prone to do, I became quickly exhausted and discouraged. I caught sight of myself in a mirror at the department store, and this did not help my emotions. The harsh overhead lighting revealed and emphasized every sag and wrinkle, and the fluorescent lighting gave my skin a greenish cast. A little while later we went into a beauty supply shop. The lighting in that store was bright, yet simultaneously soft and flattering. There were lights behind filtering panels on the walls, and so a soft radiance emanated from all sides instead of just from an overhead source. Once again, I looked at myself in one of the store's many mirrors, and I was amazed at the difference in my appearance. The harsh overhead light had exaggerated every flaw while this soft all around light made me look my best. As I stood there gazing bemusedly at my own reflection, the Lord touched my heart. In one of those *aha* moments I recognized the need to view my mother as being bathed in God's light.

As my mother's caregiver I had many opportunities to see her in less than flattering circumstances. All of the routine tasks of grooming and bathing were no longer private enterprises for Mom because she needed my help.

Embarrassment, pain from arthritis, difficulty maneuvering a walker—all of these trials would sometimes cause Mom to react negatively. The Lord was telling me clearly that in *all* of my interactions with Mom that I was to love her with God's love—that same love that had covered the whole of my sin. No partial acceptance or love was acceptable if I chose to see my mother in the best light. My Heavenly Father had never drawn a line after which He would no longer accept me or love me. God expected me to extend to my mother the same grace He had shown to me.

Today's Scripture: *"Love is patient, love is kind. It does not envy, it does not boast, it is not proud. It is not rude, it is not self-seeking, it is not easily angered, it keeps no record of wrongs. Love does not delight in evil but rejoices with the truth. It always protects, always trusts, always hopes, always perseveres" (1 Corinthians 13:4-7).*

Day 8

Avoidance Versus Knowledge

*W*hen I was expecting our first child, my husband and I attended Lamaze classes. We survived the training well until the fateful evening that our leader wheeled in a cart that wobbled under the weight of a huge reel-to-reel projector. As the film began to roll, I utilized the strategy that had stood me in good stead at so many movies in those days before the ratings system gave sensitive souls like myself fair warning; I squeezed my eyes tightly shut. But for the sound effects of groans and occasional gasps from my fellow movie goers, I made it through without much discomfort. However, when I opened my eyes at the end of the film, I was startled by the pallor of my husband's face and the perspiration that dotted his brow. We were on a limited budget in those days, but I knew a psychological advantage when I saw it and availed myself of the opportunity to get him to stop for ice cream on the way home.

Twenty-seven years later, I found a slide show at the official website of the Alzheimer's Association (www.alz. org) that elicited in me the same avoidance response as the childbirth film had done so many years before. This time though, I knew my eyes needed to stay open so that I could better understand my mother's cognitive failure. Informing myself about the disease that was causing her brain to decrease in size and function helped me to recognize her new behaviors and misperceptions as being disease related. At this writing the slide show is available at alz.org by clicking on the brain in the box labeled, "Inside the Brain."[5]

The knowledge I gained helped me to become aware of the need to analyze my mother's mental processing and to help her to use her remaining strengths to compensate for her weaknesses. This course of action was familiar to me, because as a reading teacher this is what I did for my students. In one-to-one tutoring sessions I did not project a predetermined program of progress upon my little students' unique minds. I built upon what they could do, and each day adjusted my plans to their increasing levels of ability. For my mother, it was important that I implement the same strategies I used with my students, but in reverse. I needed to be aware of her decreasing levels of functioning in order to keep her safe and comfortable.

This ability to separate the disease process from the Mother I knew and loved was a crucial shift in my thinking. Once I gained an acceptance of the fact that her aberrant behaviors were disease related, I no longer viewed myself as the long-suffering caregiver who was putting up with her mother's difficult behaviors. I was to be a facilitator, not a dictator. I became a fellow soldier with my mother in the battle against Alzheimer's. I was on her side.

Today's Scripture: *"It is not good to have zeal without knowledge, nor to be hasty and miss the way" (Proverbs 19:2).*

Insight: Don't be afraid of knowledge. There is much encouraging news in the battle against Alzheimer's disease and related disorders. Research gives hope for the future.

Day 9

Repay Insult With Blessing

A friend of mine had a heartbreaking experience when the little dog she loved was run over by a car right before her eyes. She ran to him and reached out, but her pet bit her, and she had to wait for a vet to arrive to sedate him before he could be moved. As she told me the details of this event she paused and looked at me. "You know Linda, people do that too."

I was startled and looked at her questioningly. She said, "When we are in pain we tend to strike out at those we love." I looked down at the floor in shame, because I had been complaining to her about my mother's occasional negative words and attitude toward me.

Later that day I took my complaints to the Lord, and out of the enlightenment that came from drawing near to God, I wrote the following words in my journal:

> *When we are mistreated it is ungodly to respond in kind. It is wrong to attempt to get even. It is equally wrong to examine and enumerate the exact nature of the wrongs suffered, and thus to attempt to correct the person who has hurt us. This is the equivalent of judgmental criticism. The Bible says, "Judge not" (Matthew 7:1 KJV). We become sinners when we attempt*

to correct the wrong ourselves. "*Vengeance is mine; I will repay, saith the Lord*" (Romans 12:19 KJV).

It is ineffective to ignore the hurt. A decision to ignore a hurt dealt by another human being raises a wall between us. Ignoring becomes ignorance. We close our ears and hearts to the one who has caused harm in order to be ignorant of any additional hurt they might send our way. We cannot listen to or love someone we have decided to ignore.

Love is the only antidote for the poison of resentment. The dross of vindictive anger is washed away through acts of love toward a person who has caused us pain. This kind of love must be grounded in the sure knowledge that no harm brought to us through another human being is more powerful than God's love and provision for us. "If God is for us who can be against us?" (Romans 8:31).

When Jesus was mocked He did not say a word. "When they hurled their insults at Him, He did not retaliate; when He suffered, He made no threats. Instead, He entrusted himself to Him who judges justly" (1 Peter 2:23). Watch how Jesus responded. He committed the greatest act of love that has ever been given to humankind. He died for us, bearing our sins. And by the power of God through the Holy Spirit, He has risen for us, that we might extend His love to others.

When someone commits a hurtful act against me, it is my responsibility as a forgiven sinner to commit an act of love toward them. "We love, because He first loved us" (1 John 4:19).

A few days later I had the opportunity to test this premise when an acquaintance analyzed me carefully and utilized her insights into my shortcomings to prescribe changes I needed to make in my personality. Her mode of communication was a lengthy email. I was infuriated and decided to ignore the missive, but the memory of the Lord's guidance to me regarding how I should respond to being wronged was annoyingly recent. I prayed, "Lord, You have got to help me here. Show me how to respond." It came to mind that she had worn a suit to church the previous Sunday that she had tailored herself. She was an accomplished seamstress, and I sent her an email that sincerely praised her ability and expressed my genuine admiration for the beauty of the garment she had crafted. Her response was heartwarming. She said that few people complimented her skill and that it meant so much that I had noticed. A friendship was forged.

I found that learning to respond in love to ill treatment was difficult and like any new skill, it took practice. On the rare occasions that I was able to react in a Christlike manner to being wronged, blessings were the result.

Today's Scripture: *"Do not repay evil with evil or insult with insult, but with blessing, because to this you were called so that you may inherit a blessing" (1 Peter 3:9).*

Day 10

Patience

*M*y aunt called late one evening to ask about my mother. She closed the conversation by saying, "I will pray for you to have patience."

I barely kept myself from saying, "Oh no, please don't!" To be patient, I thought, was akin to waiting in line at the grocery store behind six people with full carts when I was already late for an appointment. I believed that patience would entail clenched jaws, throbbing temples, and escalating blood pressure. It finally occurred to me that these reactions were experienced by people who *lacked* patience, not by those who knew how to wait in a way that glorified God.

Although Alzheimer's is a terminal disease, the wait time between diagnosis and the end of life is measured in years rather than in weeks or months. The *when* and *how* of the progress of the disease varies widely from individual to individual. I came to understand that there was rest to be had in the patience of waiting, because my enforced immobility released me from the responsibility to take action. Of course I completed my day-to-day responsibilities for Mom's basic care, but I did not have to launch a rescue mission for her. If I railed out against our circumstances, the effort would yield no change and I would exhaust myself.

Mom coped well because as she entered the mid-stages of the disease, she forgot that she had Alzheimer's. She was, for the most part, content in her lack of awareness. But I needed God's grace to endure, and as I sought Him, I began to view patience as a many-faceted gift.

The patience of release: When I released my mother into God's hands, I let go the reins of my attempts to control the progress of her disease. What a relief! I provided her with physical comforts, good nutrition, daily exercise, and medication; but when she suffered a downward turn in her level of functioning I was able to release myself from responsibility and self-blame.

The patience of acceptance: There was peace in the acceptance of my mother's condition.

The patience of faith: I did not have to concern myself with issues too complicated for my limited understanding to accommodate. I could have faith in God's sovereignty over our circumstances.

The patience of hope: The Lord's presence with us was dependable. Jeremiah 29:11 came to mind again and again. God intended us good and not harm; we could trust Him and hold to hope for the future.

The patience of love: Acceptance, release, faith, and hope paved the way for love. Above all else, it was most important for me to consistently express love toward my mother. When I walked in the grace of the gifts of patience, I found myself able to serve my mother's needs in love.

Today's Scripture: *"Being strengthened with all power according to His glorious might so that you may have great endurance and patience...." (Colossians 1:11).*

Chapter Five

Abide in the Lord

Abiding isn't doing, it is being. Abiding isn't abstaining,
it is indulging. I am to indulge myself in Christ.

—Linda

I used to try and let go of Him but He never let go of me …
without my faith I couldn't survive emotionally or spiritually.
Thank you, Lord.

—Anna Ruth

ᗪay 1

I Go in the Strength I Have

Not long after Mom moved in with us, I wrote the following journal entry:

Into any crisis I bring only the resources developed before the crisis occurred. A soldier can't learn new strategies of defense while engaged in a battle; a soloist can't learn a new aria during a performance. The time for developing spiritual discipline is during the easier times of life, because during the difficult times there is no surplus of emotional or physical energy. This is something to remember, because easy times bring out the old fiddler of "The Arkansas Traveler" in me. Remember? The roof didn't leak when it wasn't raining, and so he refused to expend the effort to mend it even on sunny *days.*

Sometimes I fall to the deception that if I avoid the acquisition of spiritual discipline, then I will somehow be protected against experiencing the "hard things" in life. The opposite is true, although the enemy of my soul would attempt to convince me differently. Battles will find me whether I am prepared or not. To come deeper into the Lord and to nurture my relationship with Him strengthens me to survive and to be victorious, even when I traverse "the thickets by the Jordan," (Jeremiah 12:5).

It is God's mercy and grace that see me through hard times, and my success depends on Him alone and not on any spiritual discipline I might acquire. But if during seasons of lower stress I draw near to God, the difficult times will be so much easier to bear. "They go from strength to strength," (Psalm 84:7).

Oswald Chambers says it this way, "We presume that we would be ready for battle if confronted with a great crisis, but it is not the crisis that builds something within us—it simply reveals what we are made of already."[6]

In Judges 6:15 Gideon protests that he is weak when the angel of the Lord appears to him with a command that Gideon is to save Israel. Just as God's promise and demonstrations of His presence calmed Gideon, abiding in the Lord during the less challenging periods of life enables us to go forth in His strength when times are hard.

Today's Scripture: *"The LORD turned to him and said, "Go in the strength you have" (Judges 6:14).*

Abide in the Lord

Day 2

He Bears Our Sorrows

*A*s caregiving duties became more demanding, an aversion to seeking the Lord grew in proportion to the stress of my days. I was surprised at myself and ashamed, but I did not want to come to Jesus.

I wanted to watch a movie.

I wanted to read a good book.

I wanted a brownie. Or two brownies. Or, a brownie, some caramel corn, pizza and....

I did not want to talk to the Lord about my grief and pain. When I had a few minutes I wanted to escape from thinking about anything at all. But then I remembered the comment of a dear friend following the untimely death of her husband, "The only relief I get from the sorrow and pain is when I am praising the Lord." She voiced what I knew to be true; we can suppress pain, but there is no true escape from earthly sorrows apart from God. And so, shamefacedly, I approached the throne of grace and offered my puny little praises. Of course He accepted my offering, and the troubles of my heart were eased, but still, something was lacking.

And then one Sunday morning while getting ready for church, I thought about how reluctant I was to release my grief to Jesus. I knew I had to release sins. Many times a day

I had to say, "Lord, please forgive me." But it seemed too much to ask Him to bear my grief as well. As I prayed and released grief to Him, I could see that the letting go of my pain made a bond between the Lord and me; gratitude and love on my part, and on His part divine love and a willing desire to suffer in my place.

That evening I wrote the following journal entry:

This debt I owe Him binds me to Him, but not with resentment such as an earthly debt can engender. It is gratitude, love, and praise that are birthed in my heart in response to His sacrifice for me. Releasing my grief to Him and seeing His passion, His suffering, and His willing desire to take my pain upon himself has bound me in love to Him. I worship Him. I fall at His feet.

Today's Scripture: *"Surely He took up our infirmities and carried our sorrows ... the punishment that brought us peace was upon Him, and by His wounds we are healed"* *(Isaiah 53:4a, 5b).*

Day 3

Obey, Release, Abide

*A*n abiding relationship with the Lord eluded me as long as I struggled with obedience in controlling my tongue and with discipline in my eating habits—two sins closely related geographically (if not categorically). I felt angry and frightened as my mother withdrew from me, and although I rarely lashed out at her, my husband was not safe from my angry reactions to minor disagreements.

I fell into the trap of attempting to comfort myself with food. I had struggled with undisciplined eating for years and so I couldn't blame my loss of the nurture of a mother for this sin, but somehow I felt an extra sense of entitlement because of all I'd been through. Why did I bypass the Holy Spirit Comforter for the momentary comfort and escapism offered by food that I did not need or truly want?

For me, the answer to this question lay in a reluctance to release myself and my besetting sins completely into God's hands. I wanted to take care of these issues myself. There was a secret fear of what measures might be necessary for God to accomplish a cleansing and purging. If I could only accomplish the work through my own self-discipline, I thought I could spare myself from falling into the hands of the living God which, after all, Scripture says is "a dreadful thing." (See Hebrews 10:31.) Note the misinterpretation;

Hebrews chapter 10 actually says that those who reject God's grace are the ones who must fear the dreadful judgment of the day of the Lord. I was guilty of holding God's grace at bay while I struggled to do the impossible, and I continued to struggle until one day I placed it all at God's feet.

"Dear Lord," I prayed, *"You know that I can't control my words or my eating; I keep trying and I keep failing. I release myself completely into your hands. I cast these sins on you and I accept your grace. Forgive me for hurting your heart by not allowing you to help me. I love you. Please help me or do this for me, I can't do it myself."* God counted this release as obedience, and He unleashed His power to help me. I found myself surrounded by His grace.

Today's Scripture: *"For it is by grace you have been saved, through faith—and this not from yourselves, it is the gift of God—not by works, so that no one can boast" (Ephesians 2:8-9).*

Day 4

Hide Behind the Lord 100% of the Time!

I was learning that I needed to cast the whole of my grief and sin upon Jesus. Why was this release of all that caused me pain so difficult to accomplish?

I remembered a time when I was twelve or thirteen-years-old, my mother and I had taken a walk together and were surprised by a vicious dog. Though I was old enough to act more honorably, I grabbed my mother and placed her between the snarling animal and myself. She said later that she didn't mind protecting me so much as she objected to being immobilized by the strength of my adrenalin-fueled clutch on both of her arms as I used her for a body shield! The memory of this less than heroic action has caused me shame ever since, but at the point of need I didn't hesitate to avail myself of the maternal protection that had been with me all my life. Why, then, was I so very controlled in my relationship with the Savior who had given His life for me? Why did I hesitate to release the total weight of my cares to Him? I recognized the need to stand behind my Savior's protection not only in a crisis situation, but every day of my life.

It was pride, I think, that wanted to maintain the illusion that I could handle at least a portion of my life's stresses by myself. I definitely wanted the Lord to be nearby in case I was confronted by an attack of the world's viciousness, but I wanted to keep for myself at least some of the credit for *handling things* well.

A truth that must be reaffirmed daily lest pride be resurrected in my heart is that apart from Him, I am without merit, and apart from Him, I can accomplish absolutely nothing for the Kingdom. No treasure that will last can be gathered without my Lord's help.

Today's Scripture: *"I am the vine, you are the branches; he who abides in me and I in him, he bears much fruit, for apart from me you can do nothing" (John 15:5, New American Standard Bible).*

Day 5

Comfort in the Lord

*I*n March of 2004 my daughter got married and my mother got Alzheimer's. Of course, Mom had been displaying symptoms of dementia for months and even years, but her official diagnosis came in the wake of that trembling release and flood of emotion that giving a child in marriage brings. I found myself badly in need of comfort and strength.

Aside from my mother, the mentors in my life have been authors I've never met but whose works have taken hold of my heart and led me to a deeper knowledge of the Lord. C.S. Lewis, Oswald Chambers, and Hannah Whitall Smith have each influenced me and helped to guide my walk with God. In my grief I turned to these authors, and in particular to Smith's *The God of All Comfort*.[7]

My journal was filled with pages of self examination and sentences that began with "I," but Hannah Whitall Smith took me to task for this, saying, "It is not a question of acquaintance with ourselves, or of knowing what we are, or what we do, or what we feel; it is simply and only a question of becoming acquainted with God, and getting to know what He is, and what He does, and what He feels. Comfort and peace never come from anything we know about ourselves, but only and always from what we know about Him."[8]

My tendency was to medicate my grief by seeking escapism, but once more Hannah Whithall Smith led me to the only real comfort available. She reminded me that knowing God leads to confidence and peace, not from some mystical experience or from the warmth of a temporary emotion, but from, "... just the plain matter-of-fact knowledge of God's nature and character that comes to us by believing what is revealed to us in the Bible concerning Him."

"It is of vital importance," says Hannah, "for us to understand that the Bible is a statement, not of theories, but of actual facts; and that things are not true because they are in the Bible, but they are only in the Bible because they are true."

When I opened my Bible in search of comfort, I found Him.

Today's Scripture: *"Praise be to the God and Father of our Lord Jesus Christ, the Father of compassion and the God of all comfort" (2 Corinthians 1:3).*

Day 6

Cast Cares, Not Blame

*F*or several days I had felt a rising vexation with everyone in my path. Each member of my family was avoiding me as much as possible, and this just made me angrier. As I awoke one morning in the midst of this darkness of heart, a thought came: "I need to discover the difference between casting my cares on Jesus and casting blame on others!"

As I came before the Lord in prayer I saw that the heart hurts I'd been refusing to acknowledge were acting as irritants, causing me to respond like a cranky child to the least provocation. I saw that it was impossible for me to wear the yoke of obedience to God and to struggle against my own burdens simultaneously. We are to exchange the burden of struggle for the peace and rest that result when we accept His yoke. (See Matthew 11:28,29.) We cast our cares upon Him because He loves us and will sustain us. (See Psalm 55:22, and 1 Peter 5:7.) Once again my hesitancy to open my heart fully to the Lord had caused grief for those I loved. It was the same old delusion that I'd fallen to so many times before; the crooked thought was that if I refused to recognize the presence of grief that I could avoid its ill effects.

I knew that the discomfort of grief and pain could be a portion of the Lord's yoke for me. After all, the author and finisher of our faith was a man of sorrows, acquainted with grief (See Hebrews 12:2, and Isaiah 53:3.) The fact that Christ was familiar with His grief indicates that He did not pretend that it didn't exist. To follow His example entailed an acknowledgment of my sorrow, along with acceptance of the fact that God was Sovereign over my pain. There was peace in the understanding that the Lord was with me in my grief, and even in the thought that He had ordained this path for me. I didn't have to escape from it. I could be strengthened to walk with Him through it.

I needed to ask God's forgiveness for the harm I'd done to others while I was preoccupied with a struggle against my own burdens. A journal entry from this time reveals the release that came when I cried out to the Lord:

> *God understands. He understands everything about us. He hears our cries of pain and He cries with us. He does not excuse the sin that springs from the painful ground of all we've been through; He forgives it.*
>
> *God's love and compassion for the suffering that living in a fallen world brings to us is so complete that He sacrificed His son so that we don't have to bear the consequences of the sinful behaviors that spew out unbidden from the hurts we have received. When we acknowledge the sin and plead the blood of Christ, we are forgiven.*

Today's Scripture: *"But He was pierced for our transgressions, He was crushed for our iniquities; the punishment that brought us peace was upon Him, and by His wounds we are healed" (Isaiah 53:5).*

Day 7

Intercession

During my daughter's high school years, I felt that my prayers for her were the determining factor in whether she experienced success in whatever endeavors she pursued. This was a heavy burden to bear, and it resulted in wrong conclusions on my part. If my daughter's life went well, I tended to take credit for her success. And if things went badly for her I vacillated between self-condemnation for having failed to pray adequately, and anger toward her for having somehow sabotaged my prayers.

It has been said that prayer changes things. It was easy for me to translate this to mean that "I" change things. I was slow to learn that God alone was able to bring about the changes for which I so earnestly prayed, but that He sometimes allowed me to be a part of His transforming work in the lives of others. I wore myself out and broke my own heart as I carried loads that I was not designed to bear.

The Lord has known the number of each of our days before one of them came to be, and He is sovereign over the unfolding of the events of our lives. The weaving of the fabric of our lives is in God's hands. We can't control the workings of the loom, but we can influence the color and pattern that is visible to mortal eyes by praying God's light into any given situation.

As I ministered to my family I was relieved of the burden of making sure that the events of their lives proceeded as they *should*. I was not released from my responsibility to pray for others; Scripture says that God's power through our prayers can bring healing. The Holy Spirit power that raised Jesus Christ from the dead is shed upon any given situation as I intercede, but the work that He does occurs according to God's will and not mine.

Today's Scripture: "Do not be anxious about anything, but in everything, by prayer *and petition, with thanksgiving, present your requests to God" (Philippians 4:6).*

Day 8

I Will Never Leave You or Forsake You

A lifetime relationship with the Lord enabled my mother to accept her situation with equanimity. She truly did not understand why she had to shower at my directive, or why she was required to take a walk when I said it was best that she do so; but she submitted to these indignities with no more than a shrug of her shoulders and a wry comment or two. She had to be reminded to have a daily time with the Lord, but when I placed her Bible in her lap she quickly acquiesced.

Mom had always kept a prayer and meditation journal. When I packed the contents of her house I collected a large storage container of spiral notebooks full of her thoughts and prayers; about sixty journals in all. After she was established in her new quarters in our home, she continued to keep a spiral notebook in her lap and a pen in hand. One of her journal entries from the first year after her diagnosis reads,

> *Thank you, Lord, for my feeling as good and getting around as well as I do. Praise! Thank you again for my daughter and her husband and my wonderful living situation! A picture window to look out at nature ... I will be able to see leaves come out in the spring (if it is your will, Lord). Wonderful blessings. I so enjoy*

watching nature. Oh Lord, I deserve nothing and I have so much!

Not all of her thoughts were so upbeat, but in thankfulness or in grief of loss, she continued to turn to her Lord and God.

There is no insurance policy that will protect us from adversity. The best that human sources can provide is monetary compensation in the face of tragedy. My mother's grace, courage, and calm acceptance of her circumstances challenged me to deepen my relationship with Jesus so that when I face difficult times I will be able to rest in the Lord's strength and trust in His promises.

Oswald Chambers explains that the Christian life does not mean that we are delivered from all adversity, "But it actually means being delivered in adversity, which is something very different."[9] In the midst of the adversity of confusion and helplessness, my mother was able to rest in the fact that the Lord is faithful to care for His own.

Today's Scriptures: *"The LORD himself goes before you and will be with you; He will never leave you or forsake you. Do not be afraid; do not be discouraged" (Deuteronomy 31:8).*

"Even to your old age and gray hairs I am He, I am He who will sustain you. I have made you and I will carry you; I will sustain you and I will rescue you" (Isaiah 46:4).

Day 9

At the End of My Rope

One blustery March day I managed to make my way home from work and fell onto the couch, clutching a bag of menthol cough drops in one hand and a box of tissues in the other. I was suffering my second cold in a month's time, and I found it hard to believe that an illness not requiring hospitalization and intravenous antibiotics could wreak such havoc on my entire system. I tugged a crocheted afghan over my shoulders and huddled miserably, hoping that Mom didn't need me. I felt myself to be at the end of the proverbial rope.

My capable co-caregiver wasn't due home for another couple of hours. I knew that I should start supper, but I was afraid of contaminating the food. I thought of the stack of papers to be graded, still in my school bag. I wondered whether the cat had been fed, but I didn't want to spread germs throughout Mom's apartment by going to check. I was worried that Mom was lonely because I hadn't stopped to visit with her as usual, but I knew that she would prefer loneliness to a wracking cough and runny nose. I became aware that my eyes were competing with my nose as tears ran down my face. I felt completely helpless and upset. Somewhat belatedly, it occurred to me that I should pray. I suppose that my prayer, uttered aloud, would have been comical to anyone who overheard. In a quavering voice that ended in a sobbing wail I asked the Lord to please help me.

The first thing that occurred to me was practical, and that was that I ought to stop crying. The Lord is often very practical; I remembered that when everyone was running around in a state of high emotion after He raised the little girl from the dead that Jesus said, "Give her something to eat." (See Mark 5:43.) I stopped crying. I took some medicine for the cold. I heated a can of chicken soup and sipped it from my favorite mug. I called my husband and asked him to bring home supper for Mom. And then I fell asleep on the couch.

If I had believed that I alone bore the total burden of responsibility for the well being of my students, my husband, my children and my mother, I would not have been able to have allowed myself to rest. Blessedly, I understood that this was not true. My mind could rule my emotions, and by God's grace I had the mind of Christ. And so when my emotion buffeted heart cried out in a panic, I was able to allow myself to be calmed. I knew that even if I let everyone down, that the Lord would not.

Today's Scripture: *"But I trust in you, O LORD; I say, 'You are my God.' My times are in your hands" (Psalm 31:14,15).*

Day 10

Invisible Light

As I struggled along, doubts as to God's presence and goodness would occasionally whisper. They didn't take root because the Holy Spirit had indwelt my heart and I knew that God was with me. But one day I fretfully asked the Lord, "Why do you have to be invisible, anyhow?" I then promptly forgot the inquiry, but He did not forget, and over the next few days Scriptures and hymns I came across by apparent coincidence spoke God-breathed truth in response to my question.

While preparing a Sunday school lesson, I happened to come across the great hymn "Immortal, Invisible, God Only Wise."[10] This hymn draws analogies between light and the presence of God. A lesson from a long ago science class came to mind, reminding me that there is invisible as well as visible light. I sensed the Lord showing me, as He so often does, how something that has been created reveals a spiritual truth. I remembered that infrared radiation was first called, "invisible light", because it can't be seen but can be detected with the proper instruments. Likewise, we may not be able to see God with physical eyes, but His presence can certainly be detected through the instrument of a heart warmed by His Spirit.

A day or two later my daily Bible reading included a passage from Deuteronomy 5, which tells of the Mountain of God and of a light so bright that no one but Moses was able to look upon it. The people were terrified. I remembered that Hebrews chapter 12 tells us that we have not come to a mountain such as this, but that we have access to God through Jesus Christ.

Under the old Covenant, God spoke to the people on Earth in a way that could be perceived in the physical realm, with the five senses. The Israelites heard the thunderous voice of God, saw the holy fire, and ate manna sent from Heaven. God sent Moses who spoke with Him face-to-face, and He sent many other prophets who performed astounding miracles. He appeared through a pillar of clouds, a tower of flame, and a presence that could be seen with human eyes descending on the Temple. In those days, He warned people by appearing in a way that they could perceive in the physical realm, and yet they still refused Him and rebelled against Him.

The Lord saw that the human heart, bent toward sin, would not be persuaded to loyalty and obedience even when He appeared to them in a way that was unmistakably divine and could be seen with human eyes. And so He made a new Covenant, sealed with the blood of His son, Jesus Christ, through whom we have forgiveness. Salvation didn't come to us through the laws God gave under the Old Covenant, because we are sinful. Salvation has come to us in a person, Jesus Christ, and through the love of God for us. We can now participate in God's presence through the Holy Spirit, sent to us by Jesus so that we can have constant communication with God. We can open a channel to the Lord at any time, and with no ceremony. Perhaps the Lord does not often appear to people today in physical form because we human beings forget so quickly what we have seen, and even amazing experiences fade from memory. Can't you just hear an ancient Israelite saying, "Well, yes, I know that we ate that white stuff that fell from the sky but perhaps it was just a natural phenomenon. Maybe it wasn't really God taking care of us."

In our time, God has placed His Word in our hearts by the power of the Holy Spirit and through the blood of Jesus Christ.

Today's Scriptures: *"You have not come to a mountain that can be touched and that is burning with fire; to darkness, gloom and storm; to a trumpet blast or to such a voice speaking words that those who heard it begged that no further word be spoken to them, because they could not bear what was commanded ... But you have come to Mount Zion, to the heavenly Jerusalem, the city of the living God. You have come to thousands upon thousands of angels in joyful assembly, to the church of the firstborn, whose names are written in heaven. You have come to God, the judge of all men, to the spirits of righteous men made perfect, to Jesus the mediator of a new covenant, and to the sprinkled blood that speaks a better word than the blood of Abel. See to it that you do not refuse Him who speaks. If they did not escape when they refused Him who warned them on earth, how much less will we, if we turn away from Him who warns us from heaven?" (Hebrews 12:18-25).*

"To the King eternal, immortal, invisible, the only God, be honor and glory forever and ever" (1 Timothy 1:17). Amen.

Chapter Six

You Might As Well Laugh

I find myself looking for comic relief.
Without it my perspective would become unbearably grim."

—Linda

This is one of those times when I hardly know who I am,
where I am, or why! Well, God knows and
when He is ready He will fill me in."

—Anna Ruth

Day 1

I Am a Topic of Discussion

*I*n the middle stages of her progression through Alzheimer's, Mom possessed a happy combination of faith in God along with an innate desire to avoid all things unpleasant. These characteristics allowed our relationship as caregiver and patient to be relatively free of confrontation. Her expressions of irritability were usually mild, and consisted merely of lips pressed into a thin line along with a certain shortness in her responses to my efforts at conversation. An exception to this norm was Mom's response when I invited her to any sort of physical activity, and I quickly learned to use finesse whenever I had to request that she move from her chair for any reason. She developed a system of payback for my intrusions into her peaceful and self-directed activities of reading and listening to music. She discussed me with the cat.

It was an effective weapon. I could not legitimately respond to her comments, because after all, she was not talking to me. To chastise her or to express irritation for an innocent comment to a dumb animal would have been unreasonable. I nevertheless had trouble keeping silent, because it was when she was feeling noncompliant that she was most likely to carry on conversations about me with her feline friend.

One day I was attempting to convince Mother that taking a shower was a necessary evil. She would not be openly defiant toward me, but to Poky the cat she said, "She just bothers us all the time, doesn't she? Yes she does. She isn't happy just to let us sit in our chair and read our book, is she?"

In a handout entitled "The ABC's of Coping with Alzheimer's Disease,"[11] the Alzheimer's Association admonishes, "Your loved one's ability to change is extremely limited and will diminish as the disease progresses. This means that you will have to learn to accept your loved one's behavior and learn how to alter your expectations and reactions ... you, not your loved one, will have to change." On this occasion I chose to ignore this excellent instruction and unwisely responded to Mother's indirect complaints.

I muttered, "People who complain about their daughters to cats are not being polite."

Mom did not look at me or respond directly in any way, but she cupped Poky's furry face in her hands and leaned close to confide, "She doesn't talk nice about her mother does she? No she does not."

The expression on the cat's face clearly revealed that she agreed with my mother. I was outnumbered.

Today's Scripture: *"Be completely humble and gentle; be patient, bearing with one another in love" (Ephesians 4:2).*

Day 2

Where's the Meal?

$\mathcal{A}$s Mom transitioned from fending for herself to dependence on me as her caregiver, she was afraid that I was going to forget to provide her with meals.

Her fears regarding my reliability were not entirely ungrounded. With her detailed knowledge of my life from birth to present, Mother was uncomfortably aware that I had behaved irresponsibly on many occasions. When I lived in my childhood home, my time spent in the kitchen was strictly limited to brief appearances at dinnertime, and I had been particularly adept at avoiding after meal clean-up. I didn't learn to cook until after I married. In Alzheimer's disease more recent memories begin to deteriorate first, and so as each day passed, Mom remembered less of my current, hopefully more mature and competent behaviors. Most vivid for her were memories of me as a child.

One particularly unfortunate episode had to have contributed to Mom's anxiety. The year I turned eight I owned a pair of painted turtles named Pete and Rosie. I was heartbroken when they died of starvation, and my grief was compounded because the responsibility for feeding them had been mine. Mother must have had the uncomfortable conviction that she was in danger of sharing Pete and Rosie's fate!

Mom tried a variety of methods to protect herself. She stashed rolls of crackers around her apartment and when a meal was served would lay aside a portion of it for a snack, "... to have later." I knew that this was just a polite way of saying, "... in case you forget to bring me the next meal." Reasoning with her did not help; she would forget that I'd promised faithfully to bring her food.

Despite my knowledge that mine was the behavior that needed to change whenever there was any kind of a difficulty in my caregiver/patient relationship with Mom, I allowed this situation to persist for weeks. I always served meals on time each day, and yet Mom continued to express anxiety about her food supply. Finally, I began to place healthy snacks in clear containers with easy-open lids. These were left on her counter in plain sight. For a time I also listed the day's menus on her whiteboard so that she would have the assurance that her needs would be met. Soon her anxiety faded and her hoarding behaviors disappeared along with the plaintive inquiries about the timing of the next meal.

Today's Scripture: *"Praise the Lord, O my soul, and forget not all His benefits... who satisfies your desires with good things" (Psalm 103:2, 5).*

Day 3

Midnight Madness

*M*om moved in with us in November and when Christmastime rolled around that year, I had not yet established efficient caregiving strategies. Tasks that eventually required little thought and time seemed at first to be overwhelmingly complicated. I found sorting Mom's medications to be especially challenging and I made some memorable errors as I divided ten different medications and supplements into morning and evening day-of-the-week pill dispensers. One of my really outstanding lapses was the failure to include Mom's stomach medication in any one of the compartments for the week that included Christmas day.

Our daughter Melinda and son-in-law Brian arrived late Christmas Eve in order to spend the holiday with us. Married just a few months, they were sleeping on the foldout couch in the tiny room adjacent to Mom's apartment. At 3:00 AM Mother appeared at the doorway to Bri and Mel's room, and flung open the door. "Who is there?" she demanded. Mel and Bri were both jerked to wakefulness and, not recognizing the darkened form that loomed above them, huddled close together fearfully.

139

Melinda, a member of a generation taught from birth not to reveal personal information to strangers replied, "Who is *there?*"

This stand-off might have continued indefinitely but for the fact that Brian experienced a surge of adrenalin induced clarity of perception; probably as a result of being awakened to find an intruder in his honeymoon suite. "It's your grandmother," he explained.

Melinda came upstairs and into our bedroom whispering, "Mom, Mom! Grandma's in our room!" Melinda was wearing a white t-shirt and I am extremely nearsighted. I awoke to see a diaphanous form swaying to and fro at the foot of my bed.

I screamed. This frightened my husband who leapt to his feet, became entangled in the bedspread, and fell to the floor but immediately assured us that he was unhurt. When Melinda identified herself I muttered, "I thought it was the ghost of Christmas past." Mel and I giggled together at this as we navigated our way over her father's inert form but when I saw Mom's reason for summoning help I did not feel at all like laughing. Lacking the medication she needed to help her to maintain bowel control, she had soiled her bed and several layers of clothing. The only access to Mom's quarters was through the newlywed's bedroom, and during the next hour I stumbled back and forth with armloads of laundry. Melinda had returned to her husband's side and at one point I tripped over a chair in their darkened room and narrowly missed a fall which would have landed me squarely atop their cowering forms. As I cleaned up after Mother my own stomach began to churn and I was sick as well. Although I knew my illness to be psychological in origin I couldn't rid myself of the nausea, and I was sick the rest of the night and throughout the Christmas festivities the next morning.

From this experience I learned to keep disposable gloves, baby wipes, and diaper ointment in stock. I made myself some scented masks by rubbing a little peppermint oil onto some dust masks. Most importantly I learned to never, ever forget Mom's stomach medication again.

Today's Scripture: *"I can do everything through Him who gives me strength" (Philippians 4:13).*

Caregiving Strategies

My mother's "stomach pill" was actually a cholesterol lowering medication that had a side effect of controlling her irritable bowel syndrome. I always felt that the lower cholesterol levels in her blood may have helped her cognitively as well. There is a category of cholesterol drugs called statins that some studies have seemed to show may help in the prevention or in slowing the progression of Alzheimer's. If your loved one has even moderately elevated cholesterol levels, ask your doctor about medication to control it. It is equally important to treat hypertension, if present. As a caregiver be certain that you know and manage your own numbers for blood pressure and cholesterol as well.

Day 4

Snack Time Woes

I was standing in the hallway just outside our bathroom door when the cat came rocketing past me, leapt to the counter, and began to lap water from the leaking faucet with focused urgency. I spoke her name, but she did not offer so much as a twitch of a furry ear my way. All of her attention was centered upon satisfying an apparently overwhelming thirst.

I gazed at her a few moments, then shrugged my shoulders and walked away. I lived with a farmer, a 17-year-old, and an Alzheimer patient. I was used to unusual occurrences.

Awhile later I was working in the kitchen when I noticed a chunk of cheese lying on the floor. Puzzled, I picked it up and examined it more closely. It had been broken from the layered slices of jalapeno cheese that my husband enjoyed on sandwiches. There were two bites taken from the cheese, one clearly human. The other, smaller bite could very well have been removed by a cat. Mom had evidently sampled the cheese and finding it too spicy, she either offered it to the cat or perhaps Poky removed it from the trash. Our pet's insatiable thirst was explained.

Poor Mom was still foraging for snacks to her liking. I felt compassion for her mingled with exasperation. How difficult it must be to be dependent on others for so much, after a lifetime of independence. I vowed to do a better job planning healthy and appetizing meals and snacks for her. I also needed to be sure she felt as though she had freedom to choose what she would like to eat. And, I put the jalapeno cheese in the very back of a bottom shelf in the refrigerator.

Today's Scripture: *"I am the LORD your God, who brought you up out of Egypt. Open wide your mouth and I will fill it"* *(Psalm 81:10).*

$\mathcal{C}$*aregiving* $\mathcal{S}$*trategy*

Some Alzheimer patients in the early to mid-stages of the disease retain the ability to read and comprehend written directions. Examples of how written directives worked well as a management strategy were the small signs that I placed throughout Mom's apartment. These included reminders not to let the cat go outside, the date and day's events written on a whiteboard within her line of vision when she sat in her chair, and a reminder to turn out the bathroom light. We solved the worry of her finding something in our refrigerator that would not be good for her (or the cat) to eat by placing a sign on the closed kitchen door requesting that she not enter when we weren't around. It worked.

Day 5

Nine Patch Variation

$\mathcal{E}$ ach morning I went to Mom's room to carry out a number of small chores. I adjusted the heater, made coffee, fed the cat, and raised the blinds to let in the morning sunshine. Mom was usually still in bed when I performed these small ministrations, and one day I noticed she was lying there with a big smile on her face. I looked at her inquiringly, wanting to know what had amused her. She said, "You know, when I go to Heaven they'll ask me my name, and I'll just say, 'Nine Patch Variation.'"

I was still learning not to chastise or remonstrate with Mom when her comments were inappropriate, but this was a bit much. My lack of expertise as a caregiver immediately was revealed by my reaction. Rather than simply keeping a straight face while tactfully questioning her a bit further, my mouth fell open; I stared at her incredulously and said, "HUH?"

She was not disturbed by my response. "Well," she said, "I lay here under this quilt my Mama made, and I see that it is a nine patch variation."

I nodded. Her mother had indeed made the quilt and I could see that it was a nine patch.

"Then," she continued, "I get up and go into the other room. I look back in here and I see my quilt. Nine patch variation nine patch variation nine patch variation!"

I nodded again. The rhythm and cadence of the words were beginning to penetrate and I could almost see what she meant. I waited, but no further explanation was forthcoming. Mother was happy and giggled a bit at the bemused look on my face.

I could have very effectively robbed Mom of the childish joy she was expressing and I prayed for grace to refrain from telling her to cut it out. It was so hard for me to allow her to exhibit the effects of her disease when I was never free of the grief I felt over the loss of her ability to mother me. However, on this occasion I managed to smile with her and to go about my day, leaving her to enjoy her delight in the metrical phrase that described her quilt.

But for me a few more steps of logic were needed between repeating a rhythmic phrase and asking St. Peter to enter one's name in his book as "Nine Patch Variation!"

Today's Scripture: *"A cheerful heart is good medicine"* *(Proverbs 17:22).*

145

Day 6

Good Cop, Bad Cop

*B*efore these present days of such graphic pseudo-reality on television, my husband and I enjoyed watching programs portraying law enforcement agents as they solved crimes. We would laugh at the *good cop/bad cop* method of interrogation employed by the characters on our favorite shows. When an offender refused to provide needed information, a scene would often portray one of the policemen barking threats and badgering the cowering criminal into a quivering mass of fear. The gentler and kinder partner would then move in and reason with the now cooperative thug, eliciting a confession.

I was the *bad cop* in the partnership of my marriage in the context of parenting. I possessed a thorough knowledge of the Biblical requirements for obedience to parental authority, and this was combined with a short temper and a quick tongue. Add to this the fact that I was a teacher and was accustomed to making my voice heard above a crowd of first graders, and you had a parent to be avoided if you'd done something wrong (or were *planning* to do something wrong). My husband was gentler, kinder, and more laid back. He disliked confrontation, and he hated being the cause of making anyone he loved feel badly. Our children learned that the noisier partner in a marriage is not necessarily the one who wields the most control, and they came to respect both my husband and me for our respective strengths. They knew that while Mom might set iron-clad rules for curfews or church attendance, Dad was the one to approach if you wanted to buy a car or needed help moving from your apartment to a house.

When I became the primary caregiver for my mother, my role as *the enforcer* did not diminish. During a time when I was temporarily on crutches because of a foot injury, there was a temporary reallocation of my responsibilities to others. However, I found that even when I was sitting two rooms away with my foot propped in the air that I was still blamed for all unpleasant disciplines inflicted upon my mother.

"Grandma," said daughter Melinda, "Mom says you have to take these pills."

"Linda says it's time for you to take a walk," declared my husband.

"Mom says I have to empty your trash now, Grandma," said my son.

I wasn't overly disturbed, because I'd learned that with authority comes respect. As long as I tempered my edicts with love and remembered my own fallibility, we were fine. However, one afternoon I overheard an interchange that caused me to finally draw the line. I'd spied a flea on our cat and had reacted with great zeal, bathing her twice, treating her with a prescription anti-flea rub, and vacuuming all the upholstery. A friend was at my house helping me with housecleaning chores when she laughed and said, "The cat is lying in your clean clothes basket."

I was horrified. Since my injury most clothes that I needed for daily wear had taken up temporary residence in a laundry basket in the bathroom for easy access. I had visions of fleas making their home in my lingerie. "Well, get her out," I called.

My softhearted, animal-loving friend said, "But she will think I'm the bad guy."

My tolerance snapped and I shouted, "GET HER OUT!!"

"Okay, okay," my friend replied.

She then turned to the cat and said apologetically, "Poky, Linda says you have to get out of there." Evicted from her comfortable bed, Poky stalked by me, fur ruffled and tail erect. She refused to give me a glance.

I played the role of bad cop even to the cat.

Today's Scripture: *"Our fathers disciplined us for a little while as they thought best; but God disciplines us for our good, that we may share in his holiness. No discipline seems pleasant at the time, but painful. Later on, however, it produces a harvest of righteousness and peace for those who have been trained by it. Therefore, strengthen your feeble arms and weak knees. 'Make level paths for your feet', so that the lame may not be disabled, but rather healed"* *(Hebrews 12:10-13).*

Day 7

Max the Wonder Dog

At age twelve, our dog Max was a beautiful German shepherd with eyes the color of melted chocolate and luxurious fur highlighted with tawny gold and black. He was one of the prettiest dogs I'd ever seen, and while I loved him, he had always managed to exasperate me. For example, he was jealous of anything, and I mean anything that robbed him of my attention. If I watered the geraniums by the front door he hovered resentfully, pushed at my legs, and tried to drink water from the watering can. If I took a walk he danced beside me, nipping at my hands and begging for attention.

Max particularly resented the lilac bush that graced the corner by the porch. The bush had been planted ten years earlier, when Max was just a puppy. During that time I gave the new little shrub a lot of attention, weeding, watering, and trimming. Max resented the bush mightily and one day I came out to find that he had chewed through one of the center branches. Max never forgave that bush. For the rest of his life he relieved himself on it every time he walked by, and when he was annoyed with me for any reason he would lie down beside it and chew on the lower branches, casting bitter glances my way.

Twice each day Mom and I took a walk around our circle drive. She leaned on my arm and I steadied her with both hands as we made our way along. This left no hand free to placate Max. For the first month she was with us, Max could not accept the attention I gave to Mom. He pranced around us and was scolded for endangering Mom. He then resorted to following us and barking loudly every three seconds, making conversation impossible. When this behavior did not win my attention, he ran over to the lilac bush and got down to serious chewing. I ignored his antics and continued to walk with Mom twice a day. Max adopted an *if you can't beat them, join them*, attitude and finally began to gamely follow us on our daily excursion. He still let go a resentful bark occasionally, but for the most part he finally seemed to accept that Mom needed me.

One chilly morning I was running late for work but hadn't taken Mom for her walk. I was attempting to finish a few kitchen chores before I left the house, and I hurried into Mom's room and said, "If you will put on your outdoor shoes, I'll take you for a walk in a few minutes." I returned to the kitchen and was finishing the task of loading the dishwasher when I heard Max give two, sharp 'alert' barks at Mom's screen door. I knew immediately what had happened. I ran to Mom's room and shouted, "Oh, no!" There was Mom, teetering along the gravel drive, nightgown flapping behind her, and wearing no coat as the first frost of the year glittered on the car windows. While I rushed around grabbing shoes for myself and a coat for Mom, Max did a fairly decent Lassie impression, tossing his head and running a few steps toward Mom and then back to me again. He was plainly saying, "Hurry up!"

As I galloped to Mom's side Max escorted me, watched carefully as I entwined her arm in mine, and with a satisfied expression supervised the remainder of our walk. Following

Max's heroic action I showered him with love and affection. From that day on he bore the vindicated demeanor of someone who was finally getting the appreciation due him. He was plainly saying, "It's about time."

"God takes care of His own in many wonderful ways."

— Pamela S. Runyon

Day 8

How Do Cows Know?

$\mathcal{M}$y husband helped me to take care of Mom despite a schedule that included a host of frustrations and challenges unique to his profession. Farming is never easy, but John often found himself alone, running an operation that could easily have kept three full-time workers busy. His father was seventy-nine and helped when he could. Our son at age seventeen lent a hand when he wasn't at school, football practice, or at work at his own job. All too frequently, John was alone as he cared for 300 head of cattle, planted and harvested grain, put up hay, and coped with aging equipment that we didn't have the capital to replace.

John, like most area farmers, possessed several pickup trucks, each with its own specialized function. He said that when the capabilities of his three ancient machines were added together they amounted to about three quarters of one good pickup. There was the diesel truck with the gooseneck trailer hitch, the hay truck with a fork for picking up big bales, and a "going to town" truck.

One autumn day, John began his day in pickup #2, because he'd discovered the day before that pickup #1 refused to go into reverse. He reached town, but pickup #2 spluttered to a stop in front of the flower shop and refused to start again. He walked across the street to the gas station and procured the help of Larry the mechanic. He called me and I brought him home. He set out again, not yet too discouraged, in pickup #3. This one broke down alongside the road and our son had to leave football practice in order to give his dad a ride home. All of this occurred while John's combine sat in need of repair in the middle of a partially harvested field of corn.

The next morning John sat down in the rickety old folding chair we kept on the back porch and prepared to put on his work boots. He held one steel toed boot to the light to better show me the dried greenish-brown substance that liberally decorated the sole.

His comment summed up his feelings about life in general during the past few days. "How," he asked, "do the cows know to put it right where I am going to step?"

I prayed that whether my husband was performing caregiving duties for a farm or for an Alzheimer patient that he would remember to turn to the Lord for help when he found himself standing *knee deep in difficulties!*

Today's Scripture: *"We are hard pressed on every side, but not crushed; perplexed, but not in despair; persecuted, but not abandoned; struck down, but not destroyed"* (2 Corinthians 4:7-9).

Day 9

Grace for the Trials

I had confidence that the Lord had been behind my decision to adopt a cat for my mother. I'd felt His 'nudge' in my spirit to provide Mom with a pet, and the circumstances surrounding Poky the cat's adoption had been blessed. However, there were days when I doubted the origin of Poky's spiritual heritage.

She was docile and affectionate toward my mother and more than fulfilled our hopes for Mom to have the companionship of a loving pet. But she was a one-person cat. Although she was never aggressive toward Mom, she often bit me while I brushed or fed her. One day near Christmas our adult daughter, Melinda, visited her grandmother, and made the mistake of stroking Poky's tabby striped coat. Melinda was indignant when the cat immediately sank a needle sharp tooth into her index finger, and then strutted away, offended by the unsolicited touch. It was clear that Poky considered herself to be the wronged party. I quickly bandaged the tiny puncture wound, murmuring soothing words to my offended daughter.

Poky followed her unwarranted nibble on my daughter's hand by leaping into the center of the Nativity scene display. She surveyed the small porcelain figures appraisingly and then carefully inserted her paw into the small space between Mary and Joseph. She neatly batted the sleeping infant figure from the tabletop, sending the baby flying one direction while the manger skidded under the couch. Melinda jumped to her feet and pointed her bandaged finger at the guilty animal. "Demon cat!" she shouted. Poky was shut into her feeding area in disgrace, and Melinda left for her home, still fuming about the negative characteristics of her grandmother's feline friend. I restored the Holy family to their proper places, and Mom and I shared rueful laughter over the outrageous behavior of her cat.

That evening I mused that the challenge of dealing with Poky was an apt illustration of the fact that the Lord's authorship of a given course of action does not guarantee that there will be no difficulties. When I chose to bring my mother to live with us, I was naïve and there were surprises along the way—the least of which was being forced to deal with a snooty cat. But I remembered the comfort offered me by the classic Christian poem by Annie Johnson Flint:[12]

What God Hath Promised

God hath not promised skies always blue,

Flower strewn paths all our lives through;

God hath not promised sun without rain,

Joy without sorrow, peace without pain.

But God hath promised strength for the day,

Rest for the labor, light for the way,

Grace for the trials, help from above,

Unfailing sympathy, undying love.

In all of our trials large and small, God is present with us.

Day 10

The Naughty List

Although I cut my work schedule so that I would have more time to spend at home; I did not quit teaching altogether. We hired respite care, and this allowed me to work each afternoon as a teacher in our local school's early intervention program for struggling readers.

One day just before Christmas break a colleague shared a phone number for a recording of Santa Claus. "It's just darling," she said, "and the kids all love it. You should try it." My last student of the day was a tousle headed waif named Caleb*. His teacher had told me that Caleb had an anger problem, but I had perceived it as just plain old mischievousness. For example, he regularly took my pencil when I wasn't looking and then smiled impishly, waiting for me to discover his prank. He was never openly rebellious, but he was sometimes a bit sulky or unwilling to focus on the task at hand. On this day Caleb wanted to write a story about Santa. I remembered Santa's phone number and penciled it on the corner of his homework page.

"If your Mom says it's OK, you could try to call this number tonight," I said.

The next day the phone number had been torn from the edge of the Caleb's homework sheet, and he said, "I have that phone number to Santa in my pocket. We tried to call it but he didn't answer." He scrunched up his face in a manful attempt at nonchalance, but his voice cracked just a bit as he admitted, "I think my name might be on the naughty list."

I sheepishly phoned Caleb's mother and confessed that I might have inadvertently upset her son. Blessedly, she was a woman of warm humor and after she had finished laughing she assured me that Caleb would find that Santa had remembered him with love on Christmas morning.

How often I've felt that God might not answer my call because my name could very well be on His naughty list! I had been known to sink to ridiculously infantile methods as a way to give vent to my repressed irritation with my mother. I had learned that I could never speak sharply to her or to respond in kind when she was short tempered with me because she was delicate emotionally, and the resulting upset caused more trouble than the momentary gratification of venting my annoyance was worth. But what did the Lord think of a grown woman who stuck out her tongue and waggled her fingers in her ears behind her elderly mother's back? No one but the Lord had seen . . . but that's just it. The Lord saw.

When I've sinned it is always a vast relief to remember that the Lord has made a way for me to come to Him through the blood of Christ. I know just how Caleb felt on Christmas morning when he saw the stack of packages with his name on them.

Today's Scripture: *"Thanks be to God—through Jesus Christ our Lord!" (Romans 7:25).*

* Not his real name.

Chapter Seven

A Network of Support

Help has appeared for us at every stage of this journey.
The timeliness of provision for each need has been amazing
and is one of the most comforting manifestations of
God's presence with us.

—Linda

I am blessed to be well cared for in old age. Thank you, Lord,
for your presence in my life and circumstances.

—Anna Ruth

Day 1

Cookie Delivery

My mother had lived with us for a little more than a year when I experienced several weeks of intense anger and resentment toward the world in general. I found excuses to feel anger toward nearly everyone who crossed my path, and my reasons seemed valid. However, I was aware enough to know that if the whole world looked dark while the sun was still shining that it was my perception and not the sun that was to blame.

People stopped me on the street of our little town, in church, and in the hallways of my workplace many times a day to ask about my mother. I appreciated the love and attention. Even in my dark frame of mind the caring tone and concerned attitude of those kind people was nurturing, but during this time I found myself having to bite back bitter responses as I clenched my jaw and fists to keep from acting out the anger I felt. One day though, I finally erupted when a lovely Christ-centered lady asked me a simple question.

She said, "I have some cookies for your mother from the women's group at church. Would she like a visit or would she prefer just to have you bring the cookies to her?"

I had been feeling weighted down with the duties of meeting not only my mother's physical needs, but her emotional needs as well. Those cookies suddenly seemed to me to represent the nurture and support of friends from the days when my mother was a busy and active member of her church. The transfer of the cookies from the ladies of the women's group to me seemed symbolic. "Mom once had many friends, now she only has me," I thought, and the source of my resentment was revealed. I did not want to be my mother's *all in all*. In my heart I knew that my mother's friends needed me to educate them about what was desired and acceptable, and I had rebelled against this responsibility.

They needed reassurance that although my mother did not necessarily respond with enthusiasm to the offer of a visit, she needed to remain connected to her friends nonetheless. An Alzheimer patient has lost the rhythm of the music and does not remember the steps to the dance of appropriate social interactions. My mother's negative responses were not accurate indicators of her needs for companionship and conversation. It was my job to help her friends to gain this understanding.

I had been feeling as though all my mother's eggs (or cookies) were in one basket. The basket was me and the cookies represented my services to my mother. This perception was inaccurate. I had so much support and help, and many more people who once knew and loved my mother were willing to help me; but they couldn't read my mind. I needed to initiate communication with them.

I repented of casting blame on others out of my own grief, and thanked God for people who were willing to continue to support my mother through prayers and visits. And, I thanked Him for the loving hands that had baked those cookies.

Today's Scripture: *"Carry each other's burdens, and in this way you will fulfill the law of Christ" (Galatians 6:2).*

Insight: If you find yourself bound with resentment from the feeling that you have been appointed to be the center of your loved one's universe, let yourself off the hook. God is the Provider for your loved one, and He will provide for you too.

Day 2

Pray for Me!

When my children were small I had fears about what they would do if something happened to me. I felt so very connected to them and was aware that no one else understood their needs or knew them as I did. As my mother became more dependent upon me, I began to harbor similar fears for her. What would she do without me?

One miserable morning I awoke with a high fever and found myself too ill to think clearly or to move. The predominant thought in my mind was concern for Mom. As I sought the Lord, it came strongly to mind that I should ask for prayer. I managed to email several prayer partners with my request for their intercession.

Three truths hit home during this day of infirmity. First of all, it is vital that we pray for one another whether we have been asked to do so or not. Sometimes the enemy encroaches as a trespasser and will keep the ground he's gained unless we pray. As brethren in the Body of Christ we must allow the Holy Spirit to guide our prayers for one another daily.

The next lesson the Lord had for me was the importance of asking others to pray for me when I was ill or in need. Whether from a false sense of humility or just an unwillingness to admit weakness, the inclination was to shy away from the asking. A search of Paul's letters revealed several times that Paul requests prayer as he entreats, "Pray for me...." Sometimes he even tells his intercessors specifically what to pray.

A final truth that blessed me on this day was that if I was incapacitated, the Lord would provide for my mother. A friend came and cleaned my mom's apartment and most of my house while I was sick. My daughter took a half day off work and took care of serving Mom's meals and taking her for a walk. My uncle called and chatted with Mom for the better part of an hour. My husband took her to her beauty shop appointment.

Praise God for His presence with us when we are ill, for praying friends, and for His abundant provision for us when we can't care for ourselves or those we love.

Today's Scripture: *"Therefore confess your sins to each other and pray for each other so that you may be healed. The prayer of a righteous man is powerful and effective" (James 5:16).*

*I dedicate this writing and today's Scripture
to the memory of Brad Runyon, a righteous man
who knew the effectiveness of intercession and
whose prayers were powerful.*

Day 3

The Importance of Friends

I came home bleary eyed from a day of administering reading tests to a succession of seven-year-olds. It was one of those days when I longed to escape from the pressures of teaching and caregiving, and although the supper hour was rapidly approaching and I was responsible for the evening meal, I settled into an overstuffed chair by the fireplace and switched on the television. I rarely watch TV for any extended period of time, but on this evening I immediately became engrossed in a made for TV movie. It had a beautiful heroine whose amnesia had wiped away all memory of her former life. She was engaged to a handsome hero but had terrifying flashbacks of an unremembered past. Would her abusive husband find her? Would she be kidnapped and forced to return to the terror of her former life? I was willing to sacrifice the family supper and two hours of my time to find out.

The first intrusion into my oasis of escapism came when Mother cried out my name urgently. She rarely called me unless there was a real problem and so I hurried to her room. Our two large farm dogs were both standing on their hind legs, front paws draped over the railing of the porch, hairy faces and lolling tongues pressed against the picture window. The cat lay on the window ledge in an exaggerated

166

posture of nonchalance, but I noted that she was hissing through clenched teeth each time she exhaled. Every few seconds one of the dogs would bark and the sound was earsplitting because of his proximity to the window. Mother was understandably upset to see two canines focused on her beloved pet with obvious murderous intent. I chased the dogs away with a broom, spoke a few words of comfort to Mother and to the cat, and returned to my chair by the TV.

My heroine had apparently left her fiancé and returned to her abusive husband, although she had no memory of him. How did this happen? Why had she done this? I'd missed a crucial plot twist but I was determined to catch up and I stared at the set like one who attempts to fall back to sleep in order to finish an interrupted dream. An hour passed and I once again was engrossed in my movie. At a commercial break I looked at the clock and leaped up in guilt. I slapped a sandwich together for Mother, sliced an apple, and presented it to her. To assuage my guilt over not having spent time with her I said, "Mom, when my movie is over we are going to go on our walk." Now, this is *not* the way to approach my mother regarding the prospect of physical exercise. Gentle tact and persuasive techniques are required. When confronted with this sudden news of impending energy output, Mother rebelled.

"I'm not going tonight," she said.

She often said this, but, eager to get back to my movie and not feeling patient I replied, "Oh yes you are. Just as soon as my movie gets over."

Mother flung her lap robe aside, but she had the sandwich to occupy her and I returned to the final segment of the movie. All of the twists and turns the plot had taken during the previous ninety minutes were coming together in a suspenseful climax. Would the heroine escape her now murderous husband? Would the hunky hero accept her back? One of the dogs barked and I glanced out the window. To my horror, Mother had teetered out the front door of her apartment and was shuffling rebelliously down the graveled driveway without benefit of my supporting arm. She was unsteady on her feet and never ventured out alone for fear of falling, but her anger over my having issued a direct order had propelled her outside. I levitated out of my chair and wrenched my own front door open, bounded down the porch steps, and ran to her side. I tucked my arm under hers and we made it around the driveway in record time. After resettling Mom in her chair with her supper on a tray at her side, I ran back to my TV just in time to see the credits rolling at the end of the film. I could have cried. I stood there staring at the set, fists clenched to my side. I felt like a volcano about to erupt.

I prayed, "Lord, *who can I call?*" I grabbed my cell phone and headed outdoors, walking briskly. One by one I dispensed with the names of friends who came to mind as possible candidates for the privilege of hearing me vent. I then thought of my dear friend who also happens to be my cousin. She is a social worker and has worked with Alzheimer patients. "Perfect," I thought. "She loves Mother and she knows how this disease works, and so she won't feel judgmental of Mom—or of me!" I poured the entire story out into the accepting silence of this dear woman's listening ear, and as I neared the end of my story I heard a quiet chuckle. Soon, we were both shouting with laughter as I described my emotions when I'd realized I'd missed the end of the movie.

I add "friends" to my list of survival tools for those coping with caregiving duties for an elderly parent. During this time friends have been so important to me; friends to pray for Mom and for me, and especially, friends to listen.

My friend helped me to regain my perspective, and the laughter was better medicine for my heart than any made for TV movie could've been.

Today's Scripture: *"A friend loves at all times, and a brother is born for adversity" (Proverbs 17:17).*

Insight: Do not neglect to do the work necessary to maintain your friendships. It is best to schedule a regular meeting time so as not to leave opportunities for these important interactions to chance. Phone calls and emails can also help you to stay connected to friends.

Day 4

Sandy[13]

*I*n the fall of 2003 I was still working full time, my teaching days were long, and we attended our son's sporting events several evenings a week. Our daughter had just announced her engagement, and our house was littered with bridal magazines and lists as we prepared for her spring wedding. Still in her own home, my mother had stopped cleaning or cooking for herself, and I was suffering chronic exhaustion from what was later diagnosed as hypothyroidism. One afternoon I called a friend to ask her to pray for me and found myself sobbing as I told her of all my responsibilities and worries. She recommended that I hire someone to help me with housework, but I protested. I knew that the Lord accepted me "just as I am without one plea," but there was no way I was going to allow another human being to discover that lurking under my piano were gray wads of matted fluff that merited entry in the *Guinness Book of World Records* for dust bunny longevity.

I ended that conversation with my friend with a vague intent of cleaning the house thoroughly so that I could feel comfortable hiring someone to come and clean my house thoroughly. But after several weeks went by with no time presenting itself for an in depth cleansing and purging, I gave up. I placed my pride on the altar and asked God's help. "Please, Lord," I prayed, "send someone to help me!"

The next Sunday I was sitting in my church pew waiting for services to begin, when the friend who had prayed for me stopped by to chat. She pointed across the sanctuary to a tiny lady who wore a halo of brown curls. Sitting next to her tall husband she looked even more diminutive. "That's Sandy Smith," said my friend. "She's a great housecleaner. You should call her." I looked at Sandy doubtfully. She was all of 4'11" tall and was delicately pretty. I'd pictured someone more robust. If I was going to pay to have my house cleaned I wanted someone with a lot of energy. But on my friend's advice, I made the call.

Sandy appeared at my house with a collapsible step stool tucked under one arm. She greeted me cheerfully and chatted as she got right to work. "I was at the gym this morning," she said. "I go for three hours on Monday, Wednesday and Friday mornings. Weekends I just walk a few miles or bike. And of course, I do my fifty push-ups morning and evening."

"You do fifty pushups a day?" I asked incredulously.

Our ceilings are nine feet high, but Sandy had climbed to the top of her stepstool and was energetically dusting the blades of the ceiling fan. She paused in her work and, seeming to recognize she was dealing with a slower mind than her own said patiently, "No, fifty plus fifty is 100. I do 100 pushups a day." Returning to her task she added, "And 100 crunches."

I bemusedly retreated to the kitchen and was able to give the preparation of the evening meal my full concentration while Sandy completed my cleaning chores with amazing attention to detail. Although at first I was startled to encounter such phenomena as measuring cups sorted and stacked by size and color, I recognized a good thing when I saw it and adapted quickly. When my mother moved in with us, Sandy progressed naturally into the role of "respite care provider" and her time with Mom was a blessing to us all. She was a precious gift from the Lord to us, but if I had not released my pride and sought out help, I would have missed the blessing of Sandy.

Today's Scripture: *"Ask and it will be given to you; seek and you will find; knock and the door will be opened to you. For everyone who asks receives; he who seeks finds; and to him who knocks, the door will be opened. Which of you, if his son asks for bread, will give him a stone? Or if he asks for a fish, will give him a snake? If you, then, though you are evil, know how to give good gifts to your children, how much more will your Father in heaven give good gifts to those who ask Him!"* (Matthew 7:7-11).

Insight: Pray to be blessed with the humility necessary to ask for help when you need it.

Caregiving Strategy

Contact your state's Department on Aging or your local area's Agency on Aging to obtain information on services available to the elderly.

Day 5

John and Amy[14]

When my mother broke her shoulder I was new to caregiving and was a complete novice when it came to coping with sudden injuries, seeing a loved one in pain, or responding appropriately in an emergency situation. The only thing I remembered to do correctly on the night that Mom fell was to pray, and those prayers were answered when my husband's sister Amy answered my panicked phone call. Amy is an RN, and both she and her husband John are emergency workers. They arrived to find me crouched next to my mother, afraid to touch her for fear of causing her pain. At 6'5", John is a gentle giant of a man. His movements were calm and sure, his voice soothing, and I felt better the moment he walked in the door. But it was Amy's love for my mother that brought tears of gratitude to my eyes. As she made a thorough examination of the injury, her expertise was reassuring and I will never forget the gentle strength she displayed as she wrapped her arms around Mom when it was time to help her to a sitting position. She kept hold of Mom's hand and explained each step of the process they would undergo in order to help her to stand up. And when Mom cried out in pain I saw such compassion in Amy's eyes.

I knew that the empathy and love John and Amy exhibited wasn't reserved just for personal acquaintances. Since they were family members, people connected me with them and I'd often been stopped on the street in order to receive second hand compliments. I would hear what good care Amy took of someone's aunt or father or child when they were hospitalized, and on one notable occasion an entire group of elderly ladies stopped me to tell me how much they loved John. One of their number had hurt her knee while in a water aerobics class. John's efficient rescue and strong arms had made quite an impression.

God's Word tells us that in all our distress, He too is distressed (Isaiah 63:9), and we know that His compassion is great for us when we experience physical suffering. Each of us has special gifts and is used by the Lord uniquely, but it seems to me that those who are anointed to care for people who are in pain are especially close to the heart of God. What reassurance there is in knowing that there are people like John and Amy who can express God's healing comfort and strength to us when we are in pain.

Today's Scripture: *"Now to each one the manifestation of the Spirit is given for the common good. To one there is given through the Spirit the message of wisdom, to another the message of knowledge by means of the same Spirit, to another faith by the same Spirit, to another gifts of healing"* *(1 Corinthians 12:7-9).*

Insight: God graciously provides for our needs when we are ill or in pain.

Day 6

The Alzheimer's Association

*W*hen I was writing this book I followed a carefully planned outline. I worked on the writing of each devotion for an hour or two every evening, and when I completed the day's assignment, I would end my writing session by previewing the topic for the next day's work. This allowed me to think and pray about the next evening's subject matter, and gave me time to gather resources as needed. On the morning of the day I was to write about the Alzheimer's Association, I received my *Memory Matters Newsletter*[15] from the Alzheimer's Association -- Heart of America Chapter. Thinking of the topic for that night's writing session, I smiled. The newsletter's timely arrival was an apt illustration of how this organization has been there for me exactly at the times I needed it most throughout my mother's illness. However, when I saw that the subject of the newsletter's opening article was "One Disease—Several Means of Support", I really was amazed. I had received information on ways to find support through the Alzheimer's Association on the very day that I was scheduled to write a devotion on that same topic!

I had found my responsibilities as a caregiver to be wearying. The burden was not crushing, but it was constant. During the course of my mother's illness there

175

was no closure and no clean break; just an ongoing weight of responsibility along with a dread of the final blow of her death. The support group meetings that I was able to attend provided me with the information and help I needed. As the newsletter I received that day said:

Support group members report many benefits including:

—Understanding the behavior of the individual with Alzheimer's.

—Receiving validation for negative or ambivalent feelings.

—Feeling "I'm not alone" and receiving emotional support.

—Learning specific strategies to handle their loved one's behavior.

—Receiving encouragement to maintain or regain their personal lives.

It was a remarkable coincidence to receive such a timely newsletter on a day when I needed the exact information it contained. When we as Christians trace such *coincidences* to their source we find a Father's compassion, a Savior's love, and the Holy Spirit's readiness to instruct us in the way we should go. I had once again received His reassurance that He was very present with me in my every challenge as a caregiver.

Today's Scripture: *"This is what the LORD says—your Redeemer, the Holy One of Israel: I am the LORD your God, who teaches you what is best for you, who directs you in the way you should go" (Isaiah 48:17).*

Insight: When someone close to you is diagnosed with Alzheimer's disease, you need information, guidance, and emotional support. The Alzheimer's Association provides all of this and more. Visit the association's web site at www. alzheimers.org

Day 7

Preparing for Life After Alzheimer's

*W*hen Mother was in the early stages of her Alzheimer's, I was not yet able to attend support group meetings regularly. I was still working hard to transition into the role of caregiver and was struggling with the grief of no longer having a mother who could actively care for me. I had not reached the level of acceptance that many of the caregivers with loved ones in later stages of the disease had attained, and at that point I lacked the stamina necessary to listen to heartbreaking stories of what others had suffered. It is therefore yet another testament to God's gracious provision for us that each of the three meetings I attended during those early months of my mother's illness introduced me to support services that would provide invaluable help to me during that first year of caregiving.

The first was a session entitled "The ABC's of Alzheimer's Care." The second introduced me to services available through our State Department on Aging. At the final meeting I attended, an attorney who was an expert in elder law was the guest speaker. She answered questions with a clarity that freed me of my fears of legalese. I made an appointment to visit her in her office, and she helped me through the steps of obtaining durable power of attorney for financial and health care decisions for my mother. She explained previously incomprehensible-to-me facts about the eventuality of Medicaid help for nursing home care, and she was undisturbed when I wept through most of the session.

I left her office feeling simultaneously encouraged and shaken and when I reached my car I left it sitting in the parking space while I pulled out my cell phone to call my closest friend. She listened as I talked and consoled me when my voice broke with tears and finally she said, "Linda, you know that there will be life for you after Alzheimer's."

As strange as it may seem, this fact had not occurred to me. I had not wanted to conceptualize life without the precious gift of my mother's love, which remained steadfast even as her body gave way to age and forgetfulness. This denial of the fact of my mother's eventual death had trapped me into the feeling that the ever increasing burden of caregiving was a life sentence. Grief and hope met me hand in hand that day. Yes, I was going to lose my mother. And yes, my life would go on.

In every trial the Lord offers help for the present and hope for the future.

Today's Scripture: *"For I know the plans I have for you," declares the LORD, "plans to prosper you and not to harm you, plans to give you hope and a future" (Jeremiah 29:11).*

Caregiving Strategies

• Contact your local chapter of the Alzheimer's Association for a list of Elder Law Attorneys in your area.

• It is especially important to be certain that you or another trusted individual have durable power of attorney for health care and financial decisions for your loved one.

• Obtain a copy of your state's Department on Aging publication for information about rest homes and in-home services.

• A publication I found most helpful was entitled *A Guide for Alzheimer's Disease and Related Disorders* from the Kansas Department on Aging. Your state may have a similar publication.

Day 8

Don't Quit Your Day Job

It was mid-January and the sky had become a featureless spread of granite gray. A six inch snow had fallen atop a previous storm's remnants of compacted ice; driving was difficult, and attempting to walk outdoors was even more dangerous. My uncle called and advised, "Wear your golf shoes." Unfortunately, I did not own golf shoes.

It was the third winter that my mother had lived with us. Because of the ice, we were unable to risk taking her out of the house, and friends understandably didn't want to make a trip to the country to visit. As a result I had become Mom's sole source of company and conversation as well as her beautician. I felt depressed by the weather and oppressed by the weight of caregiving responsibilities. During the fourth week of the unrelenting cold and ice I sat down at the kitchen table across from my husband and said, "I think I need to quit my job at the school. I just can't handle taking care of Mom and working too."

After thirty-three years of living with me, my husband had developed a finely honed strategy that he utilized when called upon to respond to any comment of mine with which he disagreed. He said nothing. After thirty-three years of living with him, I knew exactly what his silence implied. Lacking the energy to pick a fight with him or even to build a convincing argument in my own favor, I left him sitting at the table and went upstairs to bed.

My depression deepened the next day as I prepared to leave for work because as usual I had to leave chores undone, and I always felt guilty when I left Mom. However, as I drove away from our house I found myself daydreaming, remembering a sleepover I had unwisely hosted in honor of my daughter's eighth birthday years before. I remembered standing on our front porch as parents arrived to collect their daughters the next morning, and the sensation of vast relief I'd felt as I closed the door after they had all finally left. Suddenly I realized why that particular memory had surfaced—I was feeling that same kind of relief as I drove away from caregiving duties.

The children I worked with at my job refreshed my spirit, and my workplace provided an oasis of usefulness and ministry apart from my responsibilities to my mother. I finally recognized the truth that my husband had been wise enough to allow me time to discover on my own; I needed the mental and emotional break that my job provided. Even when my heart could not accept that my caregiving days were limited, I knew logically that at some point, I would no longer be an Alzheimer caregiver. I accepted the fact that it was vital for me to continue to invest in a life outside of my responsibilities to my mother.

Today's Scripture: *"What joy for those whose strength comes from the Lord, who have set their minds on a pilgrimage... When they walk through the Valley of Weeping, it will become a place of refreshing springs. The autumn rains will clothe it*

with blessings. They will continue to grow stronger" (Psalm 84:5-7, New Living Translation).

Insight: Your life is demanding and you are often tired, but stay involved in another job or in community activities. You need to continue to function in some role other than that of *caregiver.*

Day 9

Prayer and Fellowship

*A*n oppressive aspect of caregiving was the sense of isolation I felt as I waded through the responsibilities of my days. For years my mother had been my unfailing supporter and my sounding board. Her Alzheimer's had not robbed her of the ability to love me, and her love was a blessing to me still; but she could no longer be a dependable counselor or confidante.

I felt this loss keenly, and yet I believed that I should have matured beyond the time when I had needed my Holy Spirit filled mother to bridge the gap between my own spiritual immaturity and God's direction for my life. I remembered other times in my life when I had felt alone. I understood that the desolation of loneliness led me to greater intimacy with the Lord as I reached out to Him and found Him sufficient for my every need. Those were times of growth.

However, isolation from fellow members of God's family is not scriptural. God's Word tells us to pray for one another (James 5:16). We are instructed to bear one another's burdens (Galatians 6:2), and we are warned not to give up meeting together (Hebrews 10:25). In my unhealthy solitude I became overwhelmed and could no longer sort out the tangled mess of my own heart's needs.

With the Lord's leading and a friend's encouragement, I posted an invitation on our church's bulletin board to women who desired to meet weekly in order to pray together. Six women answered the call, and this small group began gathering together for an hour each Wednesday afternoon to follow a simple agenda. We opened with a Scripture, we shared prayer needs, and we took turns praying for one another. During the week we shared prayer requests via email, not limiting our intercession to our small group's needs. We prayed for our community, our leaders, and for needs of extended family members and acquaintances. These women did not replace my mother, and they certainly did not replace my Lord. They were precious sisters in Christ and we shared one another's burdens as the Holy Spirit led our prayers. This connectedness as fellow members of the body of Christ honored the Lord and helped each of us to make Him more the center of our respective lives.

Today's Scripture: *"And let us consider how we may spur one another on toward love and good deeds. Let us not give up meeting together, as some are in the habit of doing, but let us encourage one another"* *(Hebrews 10:24-25).*

Caregiving Strategy

If you don't belong to a Bible study or prayer group, seek out a group of people who will pray for you and for whom you can pray.

Day 10

God's Word

Since revealing is a spiritual thing, and because the Lord is not visible, He reveals himself to the eyes of our heart by the Word of God.

—*John Piper* [16]

The stress of caregiving was multifaceted and robbed me of any comfortable illusions I had managed to maintain regarding my own character. The combined weight of fear, grief, resentment, and physical weariness stripped away my fair-weather sweetness and revealed the mean-spiritedness that lurked under the surface of my usual *kindly-Christian* facade.

I quickly learned that the antidote for this unpleasant manifestation of my sinful nature was to spend time with God daily through prayer and meditation on Scripture. A daily time with the Lord had been my habit for years, so this really was nothing new for me. The change that occurred was that I became aware of needing God's Word like someone who has diabetes needs insulin. If I wanted to be able to be civil to people around me I *had* to have that time with the Lord. My poor husband learned that if he wanted to avoid my wrath that it was best to quickly turn and tiptoe away when he accidentally interrupted my quiet time. This necessity seemed to me to be humiliating. I understood that I couldn't operate independently from God, but after so many years of walking with Him I was chagrined that I hadn't been transformed into His likeness to a greater degree. It seemed to me that I should have become more *naturally nice* as a result of praying and reading Scripture for more than forty years. I didn't understand why a skipped day or two of Bible reading should have such a catastrophic effect upon my disposition. And yet, why was I so surprised? Jesus spoke this truth: "Apart from me you can do nothing," (John 15:5).

In retrospect I believe that God in His grace knew how much I needed to be aware of His presence with me during that difficult time, and that my irritability was a gift that helped to bring me to Him when I otherwise might have drifted away. When faced with grief I could either choose to attempt to avoid the pain or I could pray for strength to face the sorrow with God at my side. I wanted to run away. God in His grace brought me to His feet.

As Christians we have great freedom within the boundaries of obedience. A large section of the fence of safety that God has placed around His precious flock is the enlightenment that He provides through the teaching of the Holy Spirit as we read and meditate upon His Word.

Today's Scripture: *"Since we live by the Spirit, let us keep in step with the Spirit" (Galatians 5:25).*

Insight: Whatever else you may give up, do not sacrifice the daily intake of God's Word

Chapter Eight

Hold to Hope

Not sure where I am. Rural farm home. Where farm home? It seems this apt. should be mine but not true…my own furniture and cat—must be some of family's place. Next stop-Rest Home or with the Lord. He is in charge. Praise!

—Anna Ruth, August, 2007

Let us hold unswervingly to the hope we profess,
for He who promises is faithful.

— Hebrews 10:23

Day 1

Background Healing

I kept a journal of my thoughts and prayers throughout my time as a caregiver. Early on I developed an unhelpful habit of self-analysis as I attempted to bring each discomfort of spirit or heart before the Lord. Like a miner digging for lumps of coal, I thought I could uncover the source of my upsets in order to pray specifically and thoroughly over each difficulty.

It took too much time. The grief was too heavy, the emotions too complex, and the exercise of self-analysis yielded no fruit. I came to know that I was unable to comprehend the workings of my own heart, and that efforts to examine myself would yield inaccurate information because I was looking through the lens of my own faulty perspective. The purpose of my devotion time was not to know more of myself, but to know more of God. My journaling was of no value unless it helped me to conform my mind, my purposes, and my will to God's mind, God's purposes, and God's will.

I remembered a time years earlier when a coworker and I were in awe of our new desktop computers and printers. As we gazed at the marvelous new machines my colleague said in awe, "You can actually have the printer running and then go on to do work in other applications! It's called 'background printing'!"

As years went by, I came to take for granted the ever increasing capabilities of a succession of newer and more remarkable computers. However, the concept of background printing has continued to serve as an illustration of God's ability to work in my heart and mind to accomplish the resolution of hurts I cannot reach.

Just as I could set my computer's printer to do a print job and then go on to do other work while the printer ran in the background, the Lord could do *background healing*. I did not need to bring every grief or hurt to conscious thought, I had only to entrust myself into His hands.

Today's Scripture: *"He heals the brokenhearted and binds up their wounds" (Psalm 147:3).*

Insight: Whether you communicate with God through the written word in a journal's pages, in spoken prayers, or with an unvoiced cry from the depths of a hurting heart, He welcomes your prayers. It is not necessary to bring every hurt or grief to the fore in order to analyze and understand. God knows, God understands.

Day 2

Autumn to Winter

I loved the crisp air of fall with its spicy hint of approaching chill. Fall's glory is the doorway to bitter winter, and it seemed contradictory that I loved the signs of winter's approach and then so thoroughly disliked the cold when it actually arrived.

The trees were still dressed in autumn's red and gold when we awoke one morning to find eight inches of snow on the ground. Incredibly, the thermometer read nine degrees below zero. It was so horrible that I reacted with amusement; how much worse could it be? And then in the evening our electricity failed, and we sat for an hour in the cold and dark, wondering whether our call to the electric company would yield results or if we would be forced to sleep on the floor in Mother's bedroom next to her propane fueled, properly vented heater. What a glorious relief when the power returned and we enjoyed light and warmth again!

Life ebbs and flows like the seasons, and some times of life are bitter in excess of what we expected or knew enough to dread. It never would have occurred to me that we could suffer such harsh weather ahead of winter's official arrival. The unseasonably harsh temperatures caught us unprepared. The propane tank hadn't been filled nor had the winter's supply of wood for the fireplace been stacked.

I saw a parallel between this unseasonably harsh weather and my mother's illness. Just as we had been unprepared to meet a winter storm in autumn, I had never conceptualized the possibility that I would become an Alzheimer caregiver, nor had I attempted to prepare myself in any way for the daily stress and grief of watching my mother fade from view.

I was encouraged the morning following our power outage as I read Psalm 42 and 43. Some of the hardships the Psalmist mentions are being taunted by foes, living amongst the ungodly, being oppressed by the enemy, and suffering agony in his bones. And yet, the Psalmist remembers the Lord, praises His holy name, and entrusts himself into God's hands. I knew that I could follow this example. It was fruitless to attempt to escape from circumstances orchestrated for me and for my mother by the Lord; the only place to run was straight into His arms.

Today's Scripture: *"The LORD is my rock, my fortress and my deliverer; my God is my rock, in whom I take refuge"* *(2 Samuel 22:2,3).*

Insight: When life is bitter and you feel trapped in your circumstances, follow the Psalmist's example: "Put your hope in God, for I will yet praise Him, my Savior and my God" (Psalm 42:11b).

Day 3

I Will Choose the Voice I Follow

*I*t was February of the "winter-that-would-not-end" as I had come to call it. In bleak contrast to the usual fluctuating patterns of Kansas weather, we had endured snow cover and extremely cold temperatures for six long weeks. The very sameness of it was depressing.

Household chores were accumulating as I prepared for a presentation at work, and to make matters worse I began to suffer from confidence eroding whispers of doubt. Past failures paraded through my memory and I struggled to suppress an urge to relive the emotions of embarrassment I'd felt over real and imagined errors I'd made under similar circumstances in the past. I did my best not to entertain the doubts that were attacking me, but it was as though I was eavesdropping at the entryway to a frightening place and could not step away from the door. I didn't let them into my heart, but I couldn't help but overhear the negative words.

I knew that Ephesians 6:12 says, "For our struggle is not against flesh and blood, but against the rulers, against the authorities, against the powers of this dark world and against the spiritual forces of evil in the heavenly realms." It occurred to me that since the battle was against spirits that were in the air around me that it was then logical that I would sometimes overhear their taunting voices.

I was frustrated that I could yet be influenced in my emotions and reactions by those whispers of doubt after all that the Lord had done for me. I was reminded of the way that Peter had walked on water with confidence as long as he focused on Jesus. Of the apostle's doubts, Oswald Chambers says:

"The wind was boisterous and the waves really were high, but Peter didn't see them at first. He didn't consider them at all; he simply recognized his Lord, stepped out in recognition of Him, and 'walked on the water.' Then he began to take those things around him into account, and instantly, down he went." [17]

I prayed for the ability to attend to no other voice but the Lord's and availed myself of the spiritual weapon of praise. I sang praises and read Scripture, and the doubts were silenced as I looked at my Savior's face.

Today's Scripture: *"My sheep listen to my voice; I know them, and they follow me" (John 10:27).*

Insight: Lies can be disregarded when the Truth is known.

Day 4

Forgetting to Inhale

"The faith of many people begins to falter when apprehensions enter their thinking, and they forget the meaning of God's assurance—they forget to take a deep spiritual breath." [18]

—Oswald Chambers

During the last year that Mom lived alone her health declined. She probably had stopped eating well and was no longer exercising, but I was so busy with my own schedule that I missed signs that should have caught my attention sooner. By the time I became aware that Mom was in trouble, she had stopped taking her prescription medications. The first year she lived with us was a busy one as we addressed one health issue after another. She was sick for much of that time and fell twice. I did not have time to project to the future or to lapse to worriment because I was so busy caring for her.

We worked hard to balance Mom's diet and to provide her with daily exercise. We visited her wonderful nurse practitioner almost weekly until her medications and nutritional supplements were optimally calibrated to her needs. She grew stronger and her level of functioning improved. She became relatively self-sufficient once again, dressing herself and taking care of daily hygiene without my constant supervision. It was at the end of that first year, just at the time when my schedule grew easier and my tension over Mom should have begun to fade a bit that I began to experience physical symptoms of stress.

For several weeks I grew more aware than usual of my breathing. I would exhale and then fail to inhale until lack of oxygen drew my attention to the need. I considered seeking medical advice but then tried to imagine the prospective conversation with a physician who had seen twenty or thirty patients ahead of me, "Doctor, I've been forgetting to breathe."

And his possible reply, "You are doing amazingly well for someone who has stopped breathing."

I thus dispensed with the idea of medical intervention and took this problem to the Lord in prayer (yes, this should have been the first line of defense). It seemed immediately obvious that this was a problem of the spirit and emotions and not of the physical body. I felt immobilized. It was as though the part of me that was still my mother's little girl believed that if I held my breath I could stop time. Perhaps this childlike logic dictated that if the progression of time stopped, my mother's Alzheimer's would discontinue its relentless advance, and her death could be averted.

As I searched my Bible for the words "breathe" and "breath" I was comforted to be reminded that the Lord is the one who is in charge both of granting and taking away breath (See Job 12:10.) The Lord controlled my mother's life and the timing of her death, and I could trust Him. In Ezekiel the Lord says to the dry bones, "I will make breath enter you, and you will come to life," (Ezekiel 37:5). It was with a trembling acceptance tinged with both grief and joy that I allowed this passage to bring to mind the fact that my mother would be resurrected with Christ, and that I would meet her in Paradise.

When Daniel could scarcely breathe because of the vision he had seen, the angel of the Lord touched him and gave him strength (See Daniel 10:17-19.) I prayed to be filled with the breath of the Holy Spirit, and that He would grant me strength and freedom from the fear of losing my mother. As I turned to face the Lord and inhaled deeply of His presence, I found fear displaced by the strength of His Spirit within.

Today's Scripture: *"Let us fix our eyes on Jesus"* *(Hebrews 12:2).*

Caregiving Strategies

As a caregiver do you give the same degree of thought and planning to your own health needs as you do for your loved one? Evaluate yourself by answering the following questions:

- Do you get adequate sleep?
- Are you eating well?
- Have you seen a physician for an annual checkup?
- Do you exercise?

If the answers to any of these questions is, "No," please pray for God's help to remedy the situation.

Day 5

Guard the Heart

I continued to be aware of the need to guard my heart against resentment toward my mother. When she behaved toward me in a childish or rude manner, I often succumbed to the temptation to respond in kind. It was too human and too easy to connect Mom's real or perceived sinful behaviors past and present to the hardships I was undergoing as a caregiver. It was easy to cast blame.

In the midst of a time when I felt my anger toward Mom to be so justifiable, I read Joseph's words as he revealed himself to his frightened siblings in Genesis 45. Joseph's brothers had thrown him into a cistern, left him to suffer, and then hauled him out and sold him as a slave. He had to decide whether to keep his anger and his valid right for revenge, or to release his pain to God in order to be reconciled to his brothers. Because of his faith, Joseph knew that no human being can bring against us that which the will of God cannot encompass and turn to our blessing. The transformation from vengeful anger to forgiveness and acceptance that God's hand was behind the pain was heartrending for Joseph, but he said, "It was to save lives that God sent me ahead of you ... it was not you who sent me here, but God," (Genesis 45: 5, 8).

It was a sacrifice of obedience for me to release my perceptions of my mother's wrongdoings to God, and then to allow Him to grant me a different view. Some of my judgments against my mother had been held as fact for years and had actually become a part of my belief system about my world. Letting go was not easy and it was a process, not an event. But day by day as I attempted to *judge not,* it occurred to me that a metamorphosis was underway. If I looked closely it was as though I could see the formation of gossamer wings as a caterpillar body lengthened and became a slender support for the color and beauty of a butterfly. I could choose to focus on the still remaining resemblance to a caterpillar, and arrest the development of the beauty that was being born. Or, I could do everything possible to nourish the chrysalis because of faith, the sure knowledge of things that are yet to be. I could focus on the hope of promises given and accepted. I could remember that faith, hope and love abide, but the greatest of these is love (see1 Corinthians 13). Christ's death on the Cross was the expression of the love that had forgiven and cleansed me, and it was this love that I could in turn freely extend to Mom. My mother had not engineered the circumstances that caused me to become her caregiver. I reminded myself that the Lord was the one who had placed the job title, "Alzheimer Caregiver," after my name.

Caregiver's Prayer

Lord, grant me a heart of patience, gentleness, and love today, in Jesus' name I ask it. I forgive those who have hurt me. Thank you for forgiving me. Thank you for being in control. Thank you for working all things together according to your perfect will. Amen.

Day 6

Do Not Be Afraid

This verse from Jeremiah describes the characteristics of a person who is free from fear:

"But blessed is the man who trusts in the LORD, whose confidence is in Him. He will be like a tree planted by the water that sends out its roots by the stream. It does not fear when heat comes; its leaves are always green. It has no worries in a year of drought, and never fails to bear fruit" (Jeremiah 17:7-10).

All of my life I have suffered a tendency to give way to fear. At age sixteen I wrote a poem that included this verse: "I'm frightened of possibilities, A million fearful things, I'm even frightened of my fright; Why can't my soul just sing?" Mercifully, I gave up poetic endeavors soon after I penned those lines, but my struggle against fear continued. I learned to avoid newspapers and most television programs because reports of violent crimes and even the portrayal of them caused me such discomfort. The bad things that happened to other people caused me to lapse to fear for those I loved and for myself.

Over the years I learned that fear was dispelled when I looked to Jesus. As I remembered Him and recounted to myself all He had been to me and had done for me, fear receded. The most potent fear buster was to read Jesus' words and of His life in Scripture in both the Old and New Testaments. Just the merest whiff of the fragrance of His presence would bring a secret smile to my lips; I knew that I was His and incredibly, that He was mine.

The prospect of losing my mother provided fuel for the rekindling of old fear-based behaviors. I suffered insomnia. I was tense and irritable. I was walking through the valley of my mother's death, and I was afraid.

I awoke at 3:30 AM one morning during this fear-filled time, opened my Bible, and confessed my fear to the Lord. Physical or emotional pain can cause one to revert to childlike responses, and I had reacted in a childlike way to the fact that my father was dead and my mother was dying. If one's parents can die then anything horrible seems possible; and my fears had grown to encompass a growing apprehension that something might happen to my husband or children. I was afraid of being left alone in the world. As I cried out to the Lord I felt His great compassion and love. There was no blame. I felt a release and returned to bed and to peaceful sleep. The next morning I wrote these words in my journal:

> *God abhors fear because it keeps His children from hearing the comfort of His voice. Nothing can separate me from Him; by His death and by His life He has assured that I will always have His presence with me. However, the turmoil of fear will effectively stop up my spiritual ears so that I cannot hear His voice. My fear does not render God impotent, but it causes me to feel separated from Him, and how this must break His heart.*

As long as I was bound by fear, I could not hold to hope for the future. When I looked at my circumstances I was frightened. When I focused my attention on God's Word, my heart was quieted, and I could hear Him speaking once again.

Today's Scripture: *"So do not fear, for I am with you; do not be dismayed, for I am your God. I will strengthen you and help you; I will uphold you with my righteous right hand"* (Isaiah 41:10).

Insight: As a Christian your well being is not determined by the weather that beats upon your branches, but by where your roots abide.

Day 7

The Future is in God's Hands

*D*uring her first year with us Mom caught a terrible virus that the doctor said was, "...just one step from pneumonia." The paroxysms of coughing wore her out and caused intense pain in her shoulder, which had been injured in a fall. As one problem led to another, the antibiotic she had to take caused stomach upset culminating with a loss of bowel control.

I was exhausted and full of "what ifs." I lay awake nights wondering what would happen if I was forced to give up my job in order to care for Mom. At that time I was fifty-one years old with many years of teaching experience and a Master's degree. I knew that financially beleaguered school boards were forced to balance concern for students against funding shortages as they made hiring decisions. It is a sad truth of our profession that experience and expertise are sometimes sacrificed in order to keep the budget within reason. Common sense told me that once my caregiving days were over no school board would rehire me if a bright eyed ingénue freshly graduated from our nearby teacher's college could begin at the bottom of the salary scale.

As I pondered the facts of my situation I wrote:

I am blessed not to have to depend on common sense. I've been a Christian for forty-two years. I do not have to rely on a feeble human hope that what the Bible says is true; I have seen for myself how God cares for His own. He has never once let me down. I've learned firsthand the solid truth that stands behind phrases that sound clichéd on the surface; I know that God IS in control.

Against all odds my mother's health and level of functioning improved. This was unexpected, because Alzheimer's is marked by a slow but steady decline in abilities. At this writing my mother is in year five since her diagnosis, and although her short term memory has continued to decline, her level of functioning in such basic daily tasks as grooming and bathing has improved. I have been able to continue to hold my job, which provides health insurance for our family.

My peace of mind returned when I recognized that I did not have to worry about "What if ..." I had only to remember Who is!

Today's Scriptures: *"I am the Alpha and the Omega," says the Lord God, "who is, and who was, and who is to come, the Almighty" (Revelation 1:8).*

"Have I not commanded you? Be strong and courageous. Do not be terrified; do not be discouraged, for the LORD your God will be with you wherever you go" (Joshua 1:9).

Insight: God delights in providing solutions to our most worrisome problems in ways we would never have thought possible.

Day 8

For This Moment

*J*had begun to develop a *what's the use* attitude toward efforts to help Mom to maintain or improve her mental or physical capabilities. The very name of her illness inspired a feeling of hopelessness and helplessness: ALZHEIMER'S DISEASE.

This negative pattern of thinking expressed itself as follows: "Mom doesn't like to take a walk. It's not worth the hassle or the unpleasantness between us to insist that she do so."

And, "Mom wouldn't think of reading her Bible on her own. Why go through the discomfort of correcting my own mother by putting her Bible in front of her? She won't remember that she's read the Word anyway."

These things look horrible in print. I did not analyze myself or even recognize that I had slipped into this pattern of thinking.

The Lord corrected me through an example in my own life. I had always felt that reading my Bible should entail some hard work, like studying a textbook. Early one morning as I turned on my computer and opened my Bible journal file, I felt the Lord wooing me away from my note taking and journaling to a quiet and comfortable place. I felt compelled to come away from my word processor and found myself sitting in an overstuffed chair by the fireplace, preparing to simply read and enjoy God's Word. "But Lord," I said, "You know my learning style! I can't remember what I read unless I take notes!" I immediately thought of the Israelites, gathering manna just for that day's needs. In fact, the Lord did not allow them to gather more than they needed except for the Sabbath Day. I found my thoughts directed to my mother. Just as I could meditate upon God's Word without having to take extensive notes in order to save my insights for another day; Mom could continue to be spiritually nourished by the power of God's Word, even though her memory of it might be momentary.

As I approached my caregiving responsibilities from this new and hopeful perspective, Mom improve physically and spiritually. We walked daily, read Scripture together, and enjoyed long talks. I dug out her stretching exercise video and she completed the workout several days a week. I carried baskets of laundry to her for folding in order to encourage her contribution to household chores.

It is discouraging to face an enemy as relentless as Alzheimer's disease. There is a tendency to just make peace with what seems to be inevitable, and to lapse into avoidance. Sometimes fear makes a fight seem hopeless, but the Lord says, "Do not be afraid." He gives us strength to fight the good fight, just for this day, just for this hour, just for this moment.

Today's Scripture: *"Don't be afraid of them. Remember the Lord, who is great and awesome, and fight for your brothers,*

your sons and your daughters, your wives and your homes"
(Nehemiah 4:14).

Insight: The positive impact of loving interactions with one who suffers from Alzheimer's is retained on an emotional level, even when the details of an activity are forgotten.

Day 9

God Doesn't Make Messes

God has gifted us with imagination not so that we can better prepare for the worst, but so that we may gain a foretaste of the glory that is to be ours in Him.

When worries over finances, my mother's health, and our family's future crowded my thoughts, I learned that imagination could be either my enemy or my friend. Imagination became my ally only when I used it to help me to better envision God's Word. If I let my thoughts wander like an unsupervised child, I would find myself constructing possible scenarios of doom. I fell to the deception that if I anticipated the most distressing events that could possibly occur, I could in some way prepare myself and those I loved.

Of course, the fallacy with this line of thinking was that I didn't have adequate information to predict the future. When I attempted to do so with my *worst-case scenarios*, I trespassed on God's territory. Nevertheless, I continued to struggle with negative thought patterns until one Sunday morning Rev. Warren Wilson[19] shared the following story:

My mother used to embroider using an embroidery hoop. The top side would be beautiful, with lovely colors and a neatly organized design. But I was small, and when I would lean against her knees and look up all I could see was the underside of the work. It looked like a knotted, multi-colored mess. Even before Mom showed me her design, though, I knew that it would be beautiful. I knew it because her work graced our home and I'd seen her lovely designs on tablecloths and pillowcases and quilts. I knew it because I knew my mother, and I'd seen what she could do. Mom wouldn't make a messy design.

God is like this. He's up top, and He can see the "grand design." We're down here and sometimes things look like a mess to us. But if we've learned to know our Father in heaven, then we've learned what He can do. The secret is in knowing Him. To know Him is to trust Him. God has a plan for your life. You are precious to Him. He wouldn't make a mess of the design of your life. God doesn't make messes. If all you can see in your life right now is a mess, you can place your trust in Him. He can see the big picture, and He will not let you down.

Rev. Wilson's words helped me to the realization that although God could not be predicted that He could be trusted, regardless of how my circumstances looked to me.

Today's Scripture: *"Though the fig tree does not bud and there are no grapes on the vines, though the olive crop fails and the fields produce no food, though there are no sheep in the pen and no cattle in the stalls, yet I will rejoice in the LORD, I will be joyful in God my Savior. The Sovereign LORD is my strength; He makes my feet like the feet of a deer, He enables me to go on the heights"* *(Habakkuk 3:17-19).*

Day 10

The Bread of Life

Several years ago I decided to try a low carbohydrate diet. I purchased a special brand of bread in which a proportion of the carbohydrates had been replaced with substances that could not be digested, but allowed the product to retain the texture and some of the flavor of bread. It was not satisfying to me. I still craved the real thing.

Whenever I sought escape from the discomfort of grief over my mother, the Lord brought to me the memory of my dissatisfaction with the low carbohydrate bread. No matter how I tried to find satisfaction in false gods, the Lord would not allow me these counterfeit pleasures. I would have preferred to escape from conscious awareness of my mother's demise through extra hours of sleep, but the Lord gifted me with minor digestive disturbances that kept me from being able to lie in bed for long hours. I would have enjoyed the escapism of overindulgence in food, but twenty extra pounds brought for me a host of physical discomforts that could not be ignored. I was too tired to become a *shopaholic* and too lazy to become an exercise addict. One morning I awoke with these words in my mind: *If it looks like bread and smells like bread but does not nourish, it cannot satisfy.* When you feed your hungry heart from any source but Jesus, you quickly become hungry and thirsty again. Only Jesus, the Bread of Life, can satisfy the vast emptiness of the human heart. God has created you to be satisfied in Him and Him alone.

A few days later I was dusting my son's bedroom and found a letter that I had written to him months earlier. The note had been written during our school's "Red Ribbon Week" activities that had been designed to give young people knowledge about alcohol and drug abuse. I knew that as a Christian parent I wanted my son to understand the spiritual truths behind the "Just Say No" campaign. I had written the following words:

> When human beings seek satisfaction for heart hunger from sources other than God, they become entrapped in sin. Do not willingly hand yourself to Satan. He will attempt to deceive you into believing you are stronger than any substance or habit. He wants you to think that you can "handle" temptation. Like an expert fisherman Satan uses disobedience to hook his victims. We don't realize we are in trouble until we are being reeled in!

I was reminded that I must never take lightly the sinful tendency to seek my soul's fulfillment from any source but the Lord. All of my hope, trust, and strength must be found in Him alone.

Today's Scripture: *"Then Jesus declared, 'I am the bread of life. He who comes to me will never go hungry and he who believes in me will never be thirsty'" (John 6:35).*

Insight: In times of stress guard your heart carefully, lest you seek escapism rather than seeking hard after God.

Beautiful In Each Season

A lifetime walk with God enables a perception of beauty
in each season of life.

Reading through more than forty years worth of my mother's
meditations helped me to the realization that
although I may not be able to control what happens to me
as I age, I can nurture a relationship with God that will
see me through no matter what happens.

—Linda

This is such a pleasant place to live (and would be at) any time,
but especially in my later years. It is beautiful in each season.

—Anna Ruth, June 10, 2006

Chapter Nine

Introduction

*W*hen it was time for Mom to move from the house that had been her home for nearly forty years, I packed dozens of her journals into a large container. It took two men to carry it up the steps and into her new home: a box full of prayers and memories. A scientist might have been fascinated to examine Mom's writing to see how complexity of sentence composition and word choice deteriorated as her disease progressed, but I was inspired to chart her steadfast belief in God's love. This chapter is the result.

My mother went with grace into the dependence and infirmity of the disease which will eventually claim her life. As I read her journals I realized that the guidance she left behind is invaluable as a blueprint of how to age gracefully. Although there is no way to know what characteristics may have enabled my mother to continue to experience such peace and contentment even to the mid-stages of Alzheimer's disease, a study of her healthy spiritual habits may give some clues.

However, the alterations of character that occur with Alzheimer's disease have little to do with noble qualities cultivated in prior years—or lack thereof. There are heartbreaking accounts of kind and Christ-centered people who experience complete personality changes, and I know that the anger and violence I have seen other Alzheimer patients exhibit may yet express themselves in my mother as her condition deteriorates. The specific portion of the brain that is damaged is the physical basis for the individual expression of symptoms. This chapter is not meant to be a set of rules to follow in order to avoid "ungraceful" aging.

We walk by God's grace and not because of any virtue of our own, and this grace is ours through the shed blood of Jesus Christ. Our lives and our deaths are in His hands; "All the days ordained for me were written in your book before one of them came to be," (Psalm 139:16). Do not read this chapter thinking to emulate my mother's healthy spiritual habits and thus to avoid the pain of being a pain to others in old age! The only valid reason for the quest to develop holy life habits is the desire to glorify God.

Taking care of a loved one who is terminally ill causes our perception to telescope to the time when we will face the end of our own lives. This chapter is a challenge to each of us to put into practice those principles of Godly living that will make our brief time on this earth account for something of worth in God's Kingdom.

Day 1

You Look Just Like Your Mother

Thank you, Father! You do use imperfect vessels!
Thank you Jesus for the magnificence of creation and of
the human body—your love for individuals—so big a love
that you will work with and chastise and pummel and mold
to stretch us toward your perfection. Praise God!

— Anna Ruth, October 26, 1979

*W*hen I (Linda) was young and people told me how much I resembled my mother I always reacted with exaggerated horror. At thirteen I didn't want to admit that graying roots and an arthritic knee could possibly happen to me, and at age fifty I employed the same tactics of denial to protect myself against the thought that I might one day become elderly and dependent on others. The sinful flaw in this kind of denial was that it required a judgmental spirit in order to hold the illusion of immunity from aging in place. I read articles about Alzheimer's prevention and actually managed to build a case assigning blame to my mother for her disease. I did not hold my faulty judgment against Mom to God's light as I came to feel that if she had exercised more, or had weighed less or had been closer to the Lord, then she wouldn't have gotten sick. This gave me a sense of control over the fear that the same horror could attack me; I would exercise, I would diet, I would pray. It also gave birth to secondary sins of self-condemnation and fear whenever I failed to follow my self-imposed rules. I was not perfect any more than my mother had been perfect.

To add to my discomfiture, Mom's journals made it clear to me that she had diligently pursued spiritual and physical discipline throughout her life, often with good success. The "protection" of blame casting was taken from me. I asked God's forgiveness and for the ability to manifest His love and acceptance to Mom. Beyond that, I prayed for my eyes to be opened to the beauty of the Holy Spirit's work in my mother's life.

I was distressed to see my mother give way to aging and Alzheimer's, but it was apparent that she was for the most part content. A lifetime walk with the Lord had seen her safely through to a place in which she was able to rest in His provision of comfort for her. God's grace covered her, and as I read Mom's journals I was able to rest upon His grace for my own life as well. My path would not necessarily parallel my mother's, but God's grace was sufficient for me no matter what the future would bring.

Today's Scripture: *"But He said to me, 'My grace is sufficient for you, for my power is made perfect in weakness." Therefore I will boast all the more gladly about my weaknesses, so that Christ's power may rest on me'" (2 Corinthians 12:9).*

Caregiving Strategies

• Fear of aging can result in blame casting as you attempt to distance yourself from the facts of a loved one's failing body or mind.

• Your loved one is now and always has been flawed and sinful. So are you. Judge not.

• Recognize that God can and does use imperfect vessels to accomplish His perfect will.

• Pray for the fruit of the Spirit to be evident in your words and actions toward your loved one (Galatians 5:22).

ʼDay 2

Attitude of Gratitude

*Father God, my Savior Jesus Christ, Holy Spirit; Almighty
God I worship you, I praise you, because I choose to.*

—Anna Ruth, March 1997

𝒥 sorted Mom's journals and arranged them in chronological
order. I picked up the first of the long row of spiral
notebooks and began to read, and I found that my purpose
shifted away from a desire to protect myself from my
mother's fate as through her words I began to focus upon
Jesus. I was forced to conscious acceptance of the truth that
I could not change the fact of my own mortality or choose
the manner in which my death would come. However, I could
examine these records of my mother's Christian walk and
attempt to emulate the faith in God and the holy habits that
had enabled her to move into the infirmity and dependence
of old age with such grace.

Gratitude was a hallmark of each day's prayers for Mom.
At age thirty-eight, she was grateful to God for the gift of
life:

> *I wish I could put over on this page what zest I
> have for life—how thankful I am for the challenge of
> each day. I can't stop thanking God for not giving up
> on me—for choosing me to start feeling and knowing*

His will—feeling His influence in my life is such joy it can't be described. — June, 1962

At sixty she praised God for peace:

Thank you, Lord. I praise and thank you—for being—your creation of nature—this peaceful beauty. For answered prayer ... thank you, Lord—this quiet peace. —July 9, 1984

And at age eighty-one she continued to walk in the peace that passes understanding:

Lord, always knowing you have been and are ever present in my life—Peace. This peacefulness I feel at this time in life blesses me beyond expression. —April 6, 2006

Mom cultivated the pleasing-to-God habit of counting her blessings day by day. Gratitude to God was one of the characteristics of the faith walk that allowed Mom to experience peace even as her mind and her body began to fail.

Today's Scripture: *"Be joyful always; pray continually; give thanks in all circumstances, for this is God's will for you in Christ Jesus" (1 Thessalonians 5:16-18).*

Caregiving Strategy

Seek to cultivate an attitude of thanksgiving to God for His good gifts. The holy habit of expressing gratitude to God is pleasing to Him, and can be thought of as an insurance policy that protects against a negative attitude and a critical spirit.

Day 3

Perspective

All my life, when I thought I'd gotten a lemon,
I got lemonade!

—*Anna Ruth, March 2007*

y mother's determination to acquire God's perspective of any challenge she faced was a constant throughout her life. An example of this focus on the Lord was revealed by Mom's words regarding her marriage. My parents faced some challenges in their relationship with one another, as do most couples. But following several journal pages of prayers and an analysis of all that was wrong, Mom wrote:

> *In case sometime these inner probings of my mind and soul should fall into other hands or after I am gone from this earth, this I want known: that (though) Bob and I are incompatible in some things we love each other dearly and I am fully aware that if I had put forth as much effort to change myself to please him as he has to please me the results would no doubt have been astounding. I might add—I feel our incompatibility is no greater than most couples—especially in this last*

year—and do you know why? Because the Lord found the latchstring out and came in! —August, 1962

For Mom, "leaving the latchstring out for the Lord" involved a mental discipline of constant prayer as evidenced by this entry:

I choose to daily, moment by moment, reach out to my Lord and Savior Jesus Christ (in order to be) brought into God's presence; to be instructed by the Holy Spirit. March, 1997

In the second year after her diagnosis of Alzheimer's and in the midst of an allergy attack that left her with hives and uncomfortable itching, Mom sought God's purposes and perspective as she meditated on Psalm 2:

Never forget your Creator and Redeemer and praise and thank Him. Maybe even my allergies have a reason—without them my life would be so perfect I might get self-satisfied and that ruins it all if I do not give Christ the glory.—May, 2006

Faith in God spurred Mom to invite Him into every facet of her life, and thus she submitted to His molding influence of her heart and mind.

Today's Scripture: *"For whatsoever is born of God overcometh the world: and this is the victory that overcometh the world, even our faith" (1 John 5:4 KJV).*

Insight: Look for the Lord's purposes in every life circumstance.

Day 4

Failures

*Begin your commitment to Christ now and when you
stumble don't worry, start over. And don't shout, I will! Give
yourself to God and let Him do it.*

—*Anna Ruth, July, 1962*

$\mathcal{A}$s I read through Mom's journals I became increasingly
uncomfortable. Her patterns of thinking were familiar
to me because they were so similar to my own, and I shared
her idiosyncrasies and faults as well. We both fought
procrastination along with a tendency to enjoy comfort just a
little too much; and we both felt extreme self-condemnation
for these sins. I had not known before that Mom too filled
page upon page with self-analysis and resolutions to do
better next time; to be more organized, more fruitful for the
Kingdom, more self-controlled. These kinds of battles were
familiar to me. Time and again I also struggled too long with
self-analysis before I remembered to fall back into the grace
provided by the blood of Jesus Christ.

Mom understood the importance of submission to the
Lord, but she also knew what it meant to battle against the
flesh. The following journal entries illustrate both sides of
the dilemma St. Paul described so aptly when he said, "So

then, I myself in my mind am a slave to God's law, but in the sinful nature a slave to the law of sin, (Romans 7:25)."

Temptations will come to all and if we follow the flesh, disaster will follow. If we have trained ourselves to listen to His directions, all will be well.—July, 1962

I make the mistake of believing that I am just battling my own weaknesses, and thus I keep myself under constant condemnation. The dark one is taking my natural weaknesses and is using them to defeat me; not so much because I give in to the natural weaknesses, but because in doing so I then feel guilt and turn from God and convince myself that He has turned from me. This is not so.—February, 1980.

I have always resented taking counsel, have I not? Even my own. This (is) lack of discipline (and displays) lack of wisdom. God's Word tells me how foolish is he who will not heed correction (and yet) somehow God has given me a peace; my hand is in His; He has brought good out of this in spite of me. I praise Him for this quiet peace; my praise to God for who I am and where I am. I believe so I am counting my blessings—for this whole mechanism that is me—for the indwelling Spirit that is God in me. —January, 1980

My Christian faith begins with my belief that God came to Earth in Jesus (the Son of God). He witnessed, He taught, He died; shedding His blood for me, taking my sins upon himself that I might come to God. He arose from the dead and has gone to prepare a place for me. —January, 1978

Christ died so that our sins need not separate us from the throne of God. My mother learned to take her eyes off her own failures and to place her focus on the Lord. Through forgiveness by the blood of Jesus, she found peace.

Today's Scripture: *"Who will rescue me from this body of death? Thanks be to God—through Jesus Christ our Lord!"* *(Romans 7:24-25).*

Day 5

Involvement

Lord, I believe you are guiding me to vote for this particular presidential candidate...this should take care of the Supreme Court appointments and advisors. Thank you, Lord. I hold our country to you.

—Anna Ruth, November, 2000

In November of 2000 Mom almost certainly was beginning to exhibit some early signs of dementia. Less than six months later she failed the cognitive function portion of tests administered when she applied for long-term care insurance, and yet she managed to live alone and to function well for four more years. I believe that her active interest in church and community activities, politics, and even her interest in state university basketball games played a major role in extending the duration of her independent lifestyle.

On Election Day 2000, Mom filled a page in her journal debating the attributes of each presidential candidate. She recorded her prayers for guidance and prayed through to peace about how to cast her vote. At the end of these deliberations she wrote, "Focusing on God gives us direction in daily life."

I reviewed a three week section of her journal in the pages following those election day prayers and found that during that time Mom had completed the following activities: played cards with friends, baked and served cookies for junior choir members, conducted a circle meeting for the absentee president, watched the KU/K-State basketball game (and recorded a play by play in her journal), prepared Thanksgiving dinner for thirteen, gave two elderly friends a ride to a church function, and delivered Meals on Wheels. This is a partial record and does not include an extensive list of housecleaning chores completed. Her record of these activities are interspersed with prayers of every variety; intercession, petition, confession, and praise. Those prayers brought the Lord into the activities of Mom's life, and governed her thoughts and actions toward herself and toward others. A note written next to a Scripture reference in Mom's journal is telling: "Where can I give extravagant love today?"

Mom sought to live for Christ and to represent Him in all of the activities of her life.

Today's Scripture: *"You are the salt of the earth. But if the salt loses its saltiness, how can it be made salty again? It is no longer good for anything, except to be thrown out and trampled by men. You are the light of the world. A city on a hill cannot be hidden. Neither do people light a lamp and put it under a bowl. Instead they put it on its stand, and it gives light to everyone in the house"* (Matthew 5:13-15).

Insight: It is not enough to *stay busy*. As Christians, aging well involves a commitment to bring the salt and light of Christ into each activity of our lives.

Day 6

Service

*When we give our lives to Jesus our eternal life starts
right now—if we are His we should listen to Him every day
and do what His Holy Spirit guides us to do; in other words
we are to let the love that God gives us
flow out to God's people.*

—*Anna Ruth, January, 1978*

During my mother's retirement years, she was actively
involved in service to several elderly women. She
visited these ladies several times a month and often took
them to lunch or delivered quart jars of her homemade
chicken and noodles to their doors. I was interested to
discover that the seeds of this ministry had been planted
years before when I found that in July of 1962 Mom had
written, "I feel led to lend myself to the cause of some
elderly people. I am going to inquire today."

Later that same year Mom rated herself in several areas
of Christian discipline and wrote:

> *I must in every way strive to be a person who people
> would want to follow into Christianity.... It has been
> proven to me that if I forget self and strive to help others
> I come closer to this perfection.... Much improvement*

has been made in the area of my witnessing to my friends and neighbors but this could be improved by more thoughtfulness and follow-through for the sick and depressed.—July/August, 1962

Years later when freed of the responsibilities of a job and a daughter to raise, Mom utilized the extra time to put service to the Lord's interests in others into practice.

[I am to] relate to Jesus' interests in each person … and not just in people who appeal to me. If they praise me or blame me it should make no difference—I must serve until they know Jesus. It is not love for the person that should matter to me...but my love for you, Jesus. Many people show no gratitude but if our motive is love for God it will make no difference.—February, 1989

Mom taught Sunday school, led a youth group, was active in her church's women's group, and ministered to individuals as the Holy Spirit led. Her example of service challenged me to emerge from my self-centered focus on my own responsibilities and interests in order to become identified with Jesus Christ's interests in those around me.

Today's Scripture: *"You, my brothers, were called to be free. But do not use your freedom to indulge the sinful nature; rather, serve one another in love" (Galatians 5:13).*

Beautiful in Each Season

Day 7

What is Your Gift?

Eight years ago I started teaching because there was a job to be done and I was asked to do it. Today if that was my reason I would resign...I teach now because I feel that is where God wants me at this point.—January, 1978

During a time in which she was battling against a sense of inferiority to a slender and accomplished friend, Mom brought her feelings to the Lord and received this answer:

Use what you have to the fullest and more will be added.... Accept what you've been given—reading ability, spiritual gifts, prayer, and the ability to reach out to others. —July, 1962

My mother found that one way she was able to effectively reach out to others was through teaching. She brought the salvation message to a group of junior high age youth who gathered in her home each week, wisely giving over the organization of the group to the students themselves. They decided where to meet, how often, and what to study. Teaching directly from the Bible as per those young people's majority vote, she gave them basic instruction in the facts of the Christian faith coupled with her own personal witness to the power of the Holy Spirit through Jesus Christ by the grace of Father God. A portion of each meeting was spent in prayer. The students would spread out on Mom's family room floor, stretched full length; faces buried in their folded arms, and would take turns praying aloud as concerns were lifted before the Lord. Thirty years later the former members of that youth group still remember Mom's influence in their lives with gratitude. Of her service to youth, Mom wrote:

> *I feel it is important that young people have someone with them who desires to be open to guidance from God's Holy Spirit. I do want these young people to know the Bible and through it to know Jesus Christ in their daily lives. —January, 1978*

An important facet of my mother's faith walk involved discovering her unique gifts and using them to God's glory.

Today's Scripture: *"Just as each of us has one body with many members, and these members do not all have the same function, so in Christ we who are many form one body, and each member belongs to all the others. We have different gifts, according to the grace given us" (Romans 12:4-6).*

234

Day 8

Dealing With Difficult People

It is a lesson to reemphasize that other people cannot be depended on for your joy or your satisfaction in life, but that you cannot stop reaching out to them.

—Anna Ruth, December, 1979

$\mathcal{M}$y mother cried out to the Lord for help when other human beings caused her pain. Speaking of a group of people who had hurt her, Mom wrote:

> *Can I pray for these people in the right way, retaining concern over their negative behaviors but losing resentment for how they treat me? Losing resentment, period, but retaining concern for them? Dear God I ask through our beloved Jesus that you will help me to attain this.... [I must] show love, understanding, compassion, and pray [for them].*
> *— July, 1962*

As time passed, Mom's understanding of the mechanism for this practice of extending God's grace to others grew. She accepted that the grace that allowed her to approach the throne of God with confidence also enabled her to extend that grace to others:

> *Holy Spirit love allows people to be imperfect and still be loved—loved while their imperfections are most obvious—loved in a way that glorifies God.—May, 1978*

Mom was given wisdom that enabled her to bear in love with those who caused her pain as she recorded this guidance from the Lord:

> *...humans cannot be depended on for your spiritual or emotional support. They will fail you just as you fail them, so if you are to have love and peace it must be in and from me. I direct you not to clutch this love to you but throw your arms and heart wide open [becoming vulnerable] and let my love flow out to each one you touch with your life ... and you must widen your circle.—January, 1979*

As a caregiver, it was easy for me to slip into an attitude of resigned longsuffering as I dealt with my mother's obliviousness to my labors on her behalf. As I read her journals, Mom's own Holy Spirit inspired words spoke instruction to me of how I could bear with the unlovely behaviors she exhibited as a result of her Alzheimer's disease.

Today's Scripture: *"We who are strong ought to bear with the failings of the weak and not to please ourselves" (Romans 15:1).*

Caregiving Strategy

When you are a caregiver for a parent or for a spouse who has been your helpmate and has met your needs, you will have difficulty seeing yourself as the strong one. But the reality is that when a loved one suffers brain damage as a result of dementia, the caregiver moves into the position of strength. Pray to wield your strength with God's compassion and love.

Day 9

Trust Makes Obedience Possible

As usual, Lord, when I lose discipline, I totally lose it!
Forgiveness, Lord. Praise! Worship! Yes, forgiveness, Lord.
— *August, 1999*

R eading Mom's journals revealed not only her spiritual
strengths, but also her weaknesses. When I read of sin
in my mother's life I was encouraged, not by the fact that
she had been sinful; but because I could see that God had
exhibited great compassion toward her and had provided
richly for her despite her sin. I understood that this was not
the compassion of pity, because there is no excuse for sin in
God's eyes. This was God's love in action; the sacrificial love
that allowed Jesus to die so that my mother could live the
life of a beloved child of God. When I began to comprehend
God's grace toward Mom, I was helped toward greater trust
in His grace and provision for me. And this was a blessing
because I sometimes experienced difficulty in trusting
God.

It's just about impossible to obey someone you
don't trust. The Lord revealed to me that the root of my
disobedience to Him lay in my lack of trust in Him to care
for me. If I did not trust God to provide me help and comfort,

then I was in charge of providing for myself. And when I attempted to meet my own needs, I found myself looking for comfort from sources other than the Lord.

When the nature of my spiritual ill became clear to me, I sat down and began to write all of my so called valid reasons for hesitating to entrust myself fully to the Lord. I explained to Him that I trusted Him for my future with Him in Heaven, but that since His ways weren't my ways that I had a little trouble trusting Him for my present. My list of "Things I Wish Hadn't Happened in My Life" was scarcely begun when I sensed that the Lord was not pleased with me and I remembered His reply to Job: "Who is this who darkens my counsel with words without knowledge?" (Job 38:2). And once again words my mother had written years before were inbreathed with present day meaning for me:

> *Continually look for things that remind us that God is in all things we see or experience. Don't hold back from life in fear of being hurt—or of seeing or feeling things that are devastating to us. Sometimes these are the things [in which] we may find some of God's work for us.—July, 1962*

A life of victory over sin is not only possible; it is our heritage as children of God through the shed blood of Jesus Christ. The foundation of obedience is trust that the God who set the stars and planets in their places is able to orchestrate the circumstances of our lives for our good and for His glory.

Today's Scripture: *"May the God of hope fill you with all joy and peace as you trust in Him, so that you may overflow with hope by the power of the Holy Spirit" (Romans 15:13).*

Day 10

Conversations With God

*Question: Lord, how may I trust you
when I cannot see what is ahead?*

Answer: Trust that God knows the way.

—Anna Ruth, March, 1995

*I*n mid-life, my mother's daily journal entries often included questions addressed to the Lord. With her Bible open before her, she used a question and answer format of prayer in which she would record a query in writing and then would focus her mind and heart on God. Mom looked for her answers in the Bible, and thus the thoughts that came in response to her questions were backlit by God's Word. She knew that Scripture is key to human efforts to communicate with the Almighty, and that apart from the Holy Word of God there is danger of being subject to influences not of the Lord.

The timbre of Mom's writing changed over the years. Early on she spent much time hammering out the basics of her faith as she studied from an extensive reading list of Christian writings. In later years however, her journal entries were pared to brief petition for personal needs coupled with extensive prayer lists which consisted of columns of names of those for whom she prayed faithfully. She also spent more time recording what she had done each day, perhaps as a tool to help her to remember as she began to experience what may have been early symptoms of Alzheimer's. Appointments and daily responsibilities became oppressive for her. And yet this habit of daily seeking the Lord and calling out to Him for her own benefit and on behalf of others was so deeply ingrained that she continued recording her thoughts and prayers daily. At this writing my mother requires help to bathe and rarely leaves her chair without encouragement, and yet her open notebook is still on her lap and her pen is ready. She keeps a log of her days and addresses comments to her Lord such as, "Well, Lord, I guess I should go get dressed." She rarely follows through on such a resolution without my aid, but she does *talk* to God about it.

When my mother penned the question and answer I've recorded at the beginning of this reading, there really was great need for her to place her trust in the Lord because there were many trials just ahead. In 1997 she nursed my father to the end of his battle with lung cancer. Five months after her husband's death, her mother died. These events seemed to trigger a decline in my mother's cognitive functioning, or perhaps she was already in the early stages of dementia and the trauma of grief merely brought her struggles to light. In her 1999 journal she complained of difficulty thinking of simple words, but after all she had been through, she revealed the source of her ongoing comfort and peace:

I do come praising you for your presence with me— I know you are always with me, but this blessed sure knowledge and feeling is so—I can't think of adequate words—wonderful and great are inadequate. Yes, praise, worship, thanksgiving—all of these I extend to you.—August, 1999

241

My mother was not and is not afraid of the future because of God's presence with her.

~~

Today's Scripture: *"Yea, though I walk through the valley of the shadow of death, I will fear no evil, for thou art with me"* *(Psalm 23:4, KJV).*

Chapter Ten

From Death to Life

I tell you the truth, unless a kernel of wheat falls to the ground
and dies, it remains only a single seed. But if it dies,
it produces many seeds.

John 12:24

I must not lapse to self-pity, and I must not look at my own
sacrifice. There is nothing I can surrender to the Lord that
will not spring forth new life in Him.

—Linda

It is sad that we humans so often view death with sadness and
dread—the actuality is that it is a blessed doorway into
God's continual presence.

—Anna Ruth, June, 2007

Day 1

Darkness Into Light

One bitter October evening we lost our cat, Poky. We searched for her throughout the house, calling and looking in every conceivable location. Finally we took our search outside, and my husband found her body behind the garage. She had somehow escaped the confines of our home and as an indoor pet, lacked the stamina to survive the cold.

I was devastated. Poky had come to us as a special answer to prayer for a companion for my mother, and she had established rituals of interaction with each family member. She turned somersaults on our feet to greet us each morning and enticed us with loud meows and purrs when she wanted attention. She had a way of sprawling flat on her back with all four paws in the air that was simultaneously endearing and hilarious.

This loss tapped a well of grief in my heart and I struggled. Out of my own imperfect logic and reasoning, a thought came, "The will of God allowed it but the devil was behind it." This was not comforting because it gave too much credit to Satan, as though he could cause accidents the Lord might not have otherwise allowed. The Scripture that restored peace for me was Matthew 10:29: "Are not two sparrows sold for a penny? Yet not one of them will fall to the ground apart from the will of your Father." The phrase, "the will of your Father" jumped off the page at me. I was comforted to be reminded that the Lord is in control even of events that are devastating to us. Because I knew Him to be a loving God, there was great peace in this reminder that He was in control. We cannot comprehend the *why* of distressing events, but we may always find solace when we come to the Lord. It is a difficult truth that our only hope of deliverance from the pain of grief lies in the arms of Him who allowed us that grief.

Knowing that Mom would be lonely without her beloved pet, we visited the animal shelter and asked for a sweet tempered cat. They brought us a two-year-old calico with a nice personality, although she had a long nose with a black patch on the end and suffered from cat dandruff, poor girl. We decided to adopt her anyway and we were filling out forms when I somehow heard one plaintive little "mew" above all the other barks, yelps, and meows at the shelter. It seemed to pierce right through to my heart, and I couldn't concentrate on the paperwork I was completing. I said, "I heard a meow."

The shelter lady listened for a moment to the cacophony of noise all around us and then looked me over carefully. It was obvious that she thought that no one could pick out one particular animal's cry amidst all the din. She decided she was dealing with an eccentric and she spoke very slowly and clearly, "Yes. You are right. There are really quite a few meows." She was a nice person and didn't roll her eyes but she clearly thought me to be a little strange.

I put down the pen and said to my bemused husband, "I'll be right back!" I returned to the animal holding room and stood in front of a wall of cat cages, searching for the source of the cry I had heard. Finally, I pinpointed that one distinctive little meow. There she was, in a cage on floor level, in a far corner of the room, a tiny gray kitten. I got down on my hands and knees for a better look and she went into a frenzy of cat affection, mewing and pawing at the bars and purring loudly. I achieved eye contact and saw Poky's green eyes looking at me from a kitten face. The resemblance was amazing. Much to my husband's chagrin I yelled, "I've changed my mind! I want THIS one!"

The shelter caregivers had named the kitten "Bobbi" because of her resemblance to a bobcat, and we brought the little gray kitten with the tufted ears home. My mother was charmed immediately and from the onset the kitten spent her days purring on Mom's lap.

Sometimes the Lord prepares us for difficult life lessons in a very gentle way. Poky's death and the advent of a tiny kitten were vivid illustrations for me of several Scriptural facts: God does not willingly bring grief or suffering (See Lamentations 3:33;) His will flows over all that is grievous and changes darkness to light (See Psalm 18:28;) all things are incorporated into and transformed by His perfect will (See Romans 8:28;) where time and eternity touch, His will is done on earth as in Heaven (See Matthew 6:10;) we can't yet perceive what we will one day see clearly because we walk by faith and not by sight. (See 1 Corinthians 13:12.)

The Lord used this experience to remind me that He is sovereign over death. His good and perfect will encompasses every life event, even those that cause us pain. He is able to work every circumstance into conformity with His will, for our good.

I needed these reminders as I prepared to face the end of my mother's earthly life.

Today's Scripture: *"I will lead the blind by ways they have not known, along unfamiliar paths I will guide them; I will turn the darkness into light before them and make the rough places smooth. These are the things I will do; I will not forsake them" (Isaiah 42:16).*

Day 2

Death

I woke up early one morning thinking about Tucker*. Tucker was seven-years-old; a wiry little boy-child with a puckish grin. He won my heart with his mischievous sidelong glances and mirthful eyes as I tutored him in reading each day during his first grade year. Another reason Tucker managed to pull my heartstrings was that he had seen his pet cat run down by a car, and this awful experience had left him confused and in grief. Tucker was for a time preoccupied with death.

After reading a book about koala bears Tucker announced in sepulchral tones, "Koala bears die," and he turned mournful eyes to me. I could only nod in assent; his statement was absolutely true. Koala bears do indeed die. To no avail I attempted some platitudes about how much Koala bears enjoy life between birth and death. Another day we read a book about frogs. "Frogs die," said Tucker. "Everything dies." He looked at me as though hoping I would be able to prove otherwise and set his world to rights.

Blessedly, Tucker's preoccupation with death lasted only a few weeks, and he soon recovered his happy-go-lucky outlook. But I knew why I'd been thinking of Tucker. I, too, had become preoccupied with death. I had read that Alzheimer's is an incurable disease that inevitably leads to

249

death, and seeing this information in black and white had hurt. The recognition that my mother was going to die hit my heart, and I found myself thinking such cheerful thoughts as these: "My father died. My mother is going to die. And I am going to die." Like Tucker, I'd lost my comfortable illusion of safety from the unthinkable.

Everyone dies. A fragment of Scripture came to mind as I remembered that Jesus Christ came to, "Free those who all their lives were held in slavery by their fear of death" (Hebrews 2:15). I examined this passage in several translations and liked the way The Message says it best:

"Since the children are made of flesh and blood, it's logical that the Savior took on flesh and blood in order to rescue them by His death. By embracing death, taking it into himself, He destroyed the Devil's hold on death and freed all who cower through life, scared to death of death" (Hebrews 2:14-15, MSG).

Matthew Henry's complete commentary on Hebrews 2:14-15 says that because of what Christ has done for us on the Cross, "Death is not only a conquered enemy, but a reconciled friend...not now in the hand of Satan, but in the hand of Christ—not Satan's servant, but Christ's servant—has not hell following it, but heaven to all who are in Christ."[20]

Later that evening I wrote the following entry in my journal:

Jesus Christ has conquered death. His purpose in coming was to deliver me and to set me completely free. He is trustworthy and He is in control. I pray for grace and the will to look steadfastly at Him so that I will not be afraid.

Today's Scripture: *"Strengthen the feeble hands, steady the knees that give way; say to those with fearful hearts, 'Be strong, do not fear; your God will come" (Isaiah 35:3-4a).*

* Not his real name

Day 3

End of the Journey

I struggled to find a loving yet effective way of interacting with my mother as she became increasingly dependent upon me. At a caregivers' support group meeting, one woman described Alzheimer's as "aging in reverse." Perhaps this description helped some caregivers to cope with helpless or irrational behavior in their loved ones. However, I found that when I acted toward my mother as I had toward my children when they were young, she was offended and I was uncomfortable. Although many of her behaviors were indeed childlike, she was not a child.

When I did manage to press my will upon her from an authoritarian perspective, I tended to become patronizing and to act long-suffering. If my mother had turned into a child, then I had some basis for feeling that I'd been cheated of a parent. And if time had reversed itself for her, then what of all she had accomplished during adulthood? To treat her as a child was to dismiss the whole of who she was and who she had been to me: a mother, a teacher, a prayer warrior, and a friend.

The alternative was to recognize that she had struggled long with living and was weary. Her body was wearing out. This perspective left room to honor the work she had accomplished in her life and allowed her a well-deserved rest. I could serve her as a tribute to who she had been and with gratitude for the love she had given, and she did not have to endure my unspoken disapproval of her childlike behavior. I could treat her with the respect that was her due. A disease may have robbed her of the ability to think, and age could someday rob her body of the ability to move or to control bodily functions, but nothing could change who she had been and the work she had accomplished as she loved and served the Lord through 81 years of life.

My mother had not begun again. Time had not reversed. She was at the end of her journey. I prayed for grace to treat her with the respect and honor that was her due.

Today's Scripture: *"And you saw how the Lord your God cared for you all along the way as you traveled through the wilderness, just as a father cares for his child. Now he has brought you to this place" (Deuteronomy 1:31, NLT).*

This is the blessing my father, Bob Williamson, spoke over every family meal:

Dear Lord, we thank you for our many blessings. We thank you for this food, and we ask that you watch over us 'til the end of the journey. Amen.

From Death to Life

Day 4

Just a Little While Longer

Our friend Brad Runyon died October 12, 2005. At age 51 he wasted away from cancer. His death was not lovely in any way but one, and that is that Brad belonged to Jesus Christ.

In a conversation with Brad's wife Pam just two days after her husband's death, she mentioned in passing that although Brad's faith had remained steadfast, that he had suffered fear. His suffering was compounded because although Brad did not doubt the Lord's presence, he could not feel the comfort of His arms in the midst of suffering. This triggered a memory for me. I said, "When I was very ill years ago I learned that physical suffering can mute the awareness of the Lord's presence. It is as though our physical bodies make so much noise as we go through suffering that the *still, small voice* of the Spirit is hard to hear."

I learned this lesson when I was pregnant with my daughter twenty-five years ago. Severe morning sickness in conjunction with complications from a viral infection brought me to the threshold of death. I didn't walk the valley, but I was within sight of the entryway, and I didn't like what I saw. I was, in a word, terrified; and this despite a deep faith in my Savior. One afternoon my mother sat reading Scripture to me, and the words of 2 Corinthians 4:7

yielded a new-to-me truth: "But we have this treasure in jars of clay to show that this all-surpassing power is from God and not from us."

I saw my body as a fragile shell housing a precious treasure. Our physical bodies are like the alabaster vase that held the nard Mary poured upon the feet of Jesus. The vase was broken to release the perfume. Each of us is headed toward an appointment with physical brokenness because no one escapes physical death. Sometimes the process of death is painful and for just a little while, we are preoccupied with the breaking of the container, but then the fragrance of Christ flows forth as the spirit is released.

Another illustration is that of the pain a woman suffers during her labor to bring forth a child. In the midst of labor, few women are able to quote Scripture or to rhapsodize at length about the beauty of the spiritual realm. The physical experience of bringing forth the child is all-encompassing as enormous pressure from within threatens to break the fragile container of the body. As Brad struggled with the labor of dying, his occasional cries of fear and pain cost his family agony, but then came the release of death. Just as a woman's pain is over when her child is born, the breaking of our physical bodies through death releases our spirits to be at home with Christ. When comforting His disciples as His own physical death approached, Jesus said:

> *"You will grieve, but your grief will turn to joy. A woman giving birth to a child has pain because her time has come; but when her baby is born she forgets the anguish because of her joy that a child is born into the world. So with you: Now is your time of grief, but I will see you again and you will rejoice, and no one will take away your joy" (John 16:20b-22).*

255

Death is not lovely, but though we must walk through the valley of its shadow, there is no need to fear. In just a little while we will see Jesus and no one will take away our joy. Until that day we have the Holy Spirit in our hearts as a deposit; a guarantee of what is to come. We have a promise that will not be broken; grief *will* turn to joy.

Today's Scripture: *"Now it is God who makes both us and you stand firm in Christ. He anointed us, set His seal of ownership on us, and put His Spirit in our hearts as a deposit, guaranteeing what is to come" (2 Corinthians 1:21-23).*

Day 5

An In-Between Place

As a child I read a tale of fantasy that described a place between worlds, a sleepy, in-between place where nothing ever happened. As I sat in my mother's room one morning, the peace of her in-between place penetrated the static of my endless lists of things to do. I relaxed, and a pleasant sleepiness crept over me. However, my schedule's voice was loud and persistent, and it prevailed over my desire for rest. I jumped to my feet and once again engaged in my busyness, but I was comforted by that brief taste of the peace that fills my mother's days.

We spend our lives dreading not only death itself, but also the transition between life and death. I have always thought that the ideal last day of life would be to work all day ministering to others, and then to die peacefully in my sleep, having been productive to the end. I've felt a dread of becoming an elderly person trapped in her body, empty hands folded; all fruitfulness in the past. And yet a time of dependence upon others is a transition the Lord allows many of us to undergo before our final rest in Him. Since God is good and His love for us is perfect, this transition time must be for our good.

Even with my limited and earthbound perspective, I saw many blessings of the time my mother and I were able to spend together in the roles of caregiver and invalid. I was spared the shock of a sudden death and had time to accommodate my heart and mind to the fact of my mother's leave-taking. During those years my mother was blessed with solitude, peace, music, and time to read and to sleep in her chair. One day as I passed through her doorway dragging a full basket of laundry she observed my feverish efforts from the haven of her chair and said, "You know, I'm living the life I've always wanted." I did not appreciate that remark at the time it was uttered, but the truth of the matter was that the Lord had ordained a time of peace and contentment at the end of my mother's long labor for Him. I believe that my mother experienced a healing of memories and of the heart during this time. As she gazed at old photo albums she often stated that God had blessed her through life events that were painful at the time they occurred. In some instances I believe that the gaps in recall provided by her Alzheimer's allowed the Lord to do some editing.

Our lives and our deaths are precious to the Lord. Some of us go quickly, but for others the end of life song fades slowly, like a music box melody that comes to a gradual stop. The God who promises rest for the weary is able to use this winding down time for our blessing and for His glory.

Today's Scripture: *"He heals the brokenhearted and binds up their wounds" (Psalm 147:3).*

Day 6

To Be More

*M*y mother took five prescription drugs daily in addition to several over-the-counter supplements. As a result, I often found myself standing in line at the pharmacy, and during the wait I entertained myself by reading the covers of each of the magazines displayed in a rack in front of our pharmacist's counter. Predominately situated on the cover of nearly every magazine there were always headlines about organization. Since it seemed to me that life would be much less stressful if only it was tidy and organized, I often spent those enforced times of waiting in a daydream of ways that various areas of my house could be transformed into paragons of organizational virtue. None of these plans were ever carried out because as soon my wait was over I was immediately engulfed once again by all of the little tasks that made up the ordinary responsibilities of my days. Nevertheless, I nursed a fair amount of longing for a life that was uncluttered and orderly.

I suffered several unsatisfied ambitions of which *to be more organized* was just one. I wanted to be more loving, to be more slender; to be more of everything praiseworthy and good. These desires had not much to do with the actual working out of my salvation (mere longing involves no real work at all), but were based upon a desire to arrive at a place of perfection at which time no more struggle would be required.

The daily release of these longings to the Lord was a kind of death. It was difficult to lay my own self-directed quests for an appearance of perfection at the altar. I wanted to look good on the outside, and I had noticed that sometimes when we do kingdom work the housework suffers, the diet is not followed, and the redecorating is set aside for another day. With the busy schedule of a mother, wife, and caregiver, it became more difficult and more important for me to exchange the good for the best. Apart from a daily realignment with the Lord my days became filled with the frustration of attempting to *accomplish things* apart from Him.

My heart's longing for order was satisfied only through a daily, abiding relationship with God. I learned that this was not just a mental exercise or a discipline of the emotions; but rather it involved an active appropriation of the power that is ours in Christ. Putting Him first pulled the rest of my life into order and, as always, I found that when I was in right relationship with Him, I was free of longings after things that could not satisfy.

Today's Scripture: *"Why spend money on what is not bread, and your labor on what does not satisfy? Listen, listen to me, and eat what is good, and your soul will delight in the richest of fare"* *(Isaiah 55:2).*

Insight: The best organizational strategy that a Christian can utilize is the nurture of an abiding relationship with Christ.

Day 7

The Journey Home

*W*hen I was four-years-old our family moved away from the little bungalow that had been my home since birth. Situated on a scenic fifteen acres, we had called that idyllic place, "the farm." With a child's lack of understanding I pined for the big tree, my rope swing and the beautiful yard and garden we left behind. I've read that it is unwise to change a child's environment at the age of four or five because of a particular vulnerability in mental and emotional development at this age. This was true for me, because I suffered a kind of homesickness for years following that move and even now, nearly fifty years later, I experience a strong nostalgia laced with longing whenever I think of that childhood home.

Perhaps as a result of that early experience I have always hated change. I had an ongoing desire to attain security for myself in my living situation. It was inordinately important to me that my husband and I own our own home and I prayed hard until this was accomplished for us. When my mother came to live with us I learned that a portion of the great difficulty I suffered in watching her fade away physically and mentally had to do with the fact that I wanted her to stay the same. The old childhood hurt of leaving behind that which was dear to me raised its head, and I found myself thinking often of that little house on the farm of long ago. One day when I was sorting through a box of my mother's belongings I uncovered a scrap of fabric that had been used in the curtains at that old home, and I was reduced to tears of helpless longing and grief.

In prayer, I remembered that the Israelites were always traveling, never home. During their forty years in the desert, every encampment was only a temporary home. This mirrors our journey through life. Until we are at home with the Lord we are always arriving at a new place, taking a temporary rest, and then moving on. I came to a shaky acceptance of the fact that during my sojourn here I am never going to attain an unassailable physical haven of security. There is no Promised Land here on Earth; it waits for us in Heaven. The Lord gives times of rest, like oases in the desert of this journey through life, but I must never mistake a short-term respite for a permanent dwelling. This temporary shelter is where I live for now, but Heaven is my home.

Today's Scripture: *"Blessed are those who dwell in your house; they are ever praising you" (Psalm 84:4).*

Day 8

To Live Is Christ

When I was growing up, a story I heard often had to do with the sudden and unexpected way in which my great-grandfather died. He was just in his early fifties when he collapsed and died of a heart attack while leading a horse in a show ring. My grandfather was impacted by aftershocks from his father's sudden death for the rest of his life. His angst was compounded when he reached his fifties and passed the age his own father had been at his death. My grandfather fully expected to die well in advance of his sixtieth birthday. We all used to smile at his mournful comment to my grandmother each fall as he would say, "Well, Opal, I've cut enough wood to last you the winter in case anything should happen to me." Nothing ever did happen to him, and he lived to be ninety-three years old. The story of his ongoing commitment to provision for his family "just in case anything happens" was told at the gathering following his funeral; an event that finally occurred approximately forty years later than my grandfather had expected it.

I suffered from a similar malady to my grandpa's ongoing sense of impending doom when I was watching my mother fade away from the effects of Alzheimer's disease. I became somewhat morbid and introspective for a time. Perhaps because I had always been so close to my mom, it was as though my life telescoped forward about thirty years as I began to think and feel from her perspective. I didn't feel like a spectator; I felt like death was happening to me. I drove my kids crazy as I cleaned out closets and labeled boxes of family mementos, "So you kids won't have such a mess after I'm gone."

My daughter said emphatically, "You are not going anywhere for a long time yet," but I ignored her. Death had become real to me and I knew what she had not yet learned; it happens to those you love. Until she lost a loved one she couldn't really understand this fact. The timelines of our lives overlap, but they do not begin or end in tandem. There would be a terrible loneliness in this fact, but for the Lord and His promise that He will never leave or forsake us.

I knew I had a choice about how to deal with my grief over the inevitable ending of my own life and the lives of those I loved. I very much wanted to anesthetize the pain of it, and finding avenues of escape was easy to do when I turned my eyes to the smorgasbord of the world's offerings. The alternative that I eventually chose was to face the facts with Jesus at my side; to delve deeper into Him and to find, amazingly, a glint of amusement in His eye as He helped me to the realization that death truly is the doorway to new life. He delighted to share His joy with me, and I could hear Him say, "Look! I am alive! And you will someday be with Me where I am!"

When I looked into His eyes I began to comprehend the truth of the Apostle's words, "To live is Christ, and to die is gain" (Philippians 1:21).

Today's Scripture: *"If I am to go on living in the body, this will mean fruitful labor for me...Whatever happens, conduct yourself in a manner worthy of the Gospel of Christ" (Philippians 1:22,27).*

Day 9

Lay It Down

*W*hen my son-in-law Brian was in college, he navigated around campus on a motorcycle. He was well versed in the language of the road, and with stars in her eyes directed toward the handsome young art major on the motorcycle, my daughter Melinda became acquainted with terminology I'd not heard before. One day I was talking to her on her cell phone as Brian was pulling away from her dorm on his bike. I could hear the motor revving in the background as Melinda shouted a farewell; "Bye! Don't lay it down!" I had no idea what she meant and she explained, "When motorcycle riders wreck they call it, 'Laying it down.'"

It occurred to me that while *laying it down* is something any motorcycle rider in his right mind wants very much to avoid, the exact opposite is true in our relationship with the Lord. It's the paradox of letting go of what is mine in order to lay hold of what the Lord offers, and it is difficult because laying it down feels like the wrong thing to do.

Bearing responsibility for my mother required a daily relinquishment of my time that, in the beginning, just didn't feel right. Like a motorcycle rider striving desperately to keep from coming into full body contact with the pavement, I had a lot of difficulty giving up the right to keep control of my own life.

The ultimate release that is the result of going on to maturity in Christ is the laying down of our lives for His use. Oswald Chambers says it like this: "The delight of sacrifice is that I lay down my life for my Friend, Jesus. I don't throw my life away, but I willingly and deliberately lay it down for Him and His interests in other people."[21]

Today's Scripture: *"This is how we know what love is: Jesus Christ laid down His life for us. And we ought to lay down our lives for our brothers"* (1 John 3:16).

Day 10

Death to Life

During the mid stages of my mother's battle with Alzheimer's, her symptoms were textbook: lack of motivation, withdrawal from reality, and agitation in response to changes in schedule or location. I came to accept that these symptoms were not the result of a personality flaw but were the manifestations of her disease.

Sin was more apparent as the will to fight was compromised. I sometimes looked at my mother and was afraid. She had always been a better and kinder person than I, and yet she struggled with resentment against the helplessness of old age. I was the volatile child who shouted out against anything I perceived to be unfair. The injustices my mother was facing, real and perceived, were overwhelming. What would happen to me under the same pressures?

We are all sinful. I had to accept that I was not going to be able to turn over a new leaf and become sin-free. I had that in my mind to do, I think; to become so free of sin that as an old lady I would not cause my daughter to feel revulsion toward me, or my son to avoid me. I wanted to take out insurance against rejection by becoming so perfect that there would be nothing left to reject. Of course there was no program of self-improvement that could rescue me (or my children) from the fruits of my sins. We do not perfect ourselves; perfection has been purchased for us, and we attain it only by participating in the death and resurrection of Jesus Christ. During earthly life we can put to death the misdeeds of the body by walking according to the Spirit (See Romans 8:13.) At the end of mortal life we who have been made righteous by the blood of Christ are perfected in Him (See Hebrews 12:23.) Death comes first, and the dying is painful to watch and painful to endure. The process that perfects us, kills us; but we are raised to new life. I was afraid of being old and alone; confused, and in grief.

My father died in 1997, three weeks after Christmas. There is a photo taken of him at that last Christmas celebration in which he is engulfed by light. He wasn't sitting near a window and there's no explanation for the light that I can see. My father was a loving but volatile man, and he struggled against sins of the tongue throughout his life. Yet, because of his acceptance of Jesus as Lord, his sins were swallowed by victory; his spirit set free. The first Christmas following my mother's diagnosis with Alzheimer's disease, several photos showed her to be engulfed by the light from a window. I knew the Lord was telling me that at the end, there will be victory.

The life of Christ is at work in those of us who love Him and believe in Him. As we walk with Him we become more like Him. At the end of our earthly lives, all that is not of Him will be swallowed by victory. This comes, not from any good in us, but from the wondrous gift of grace through the blood of Jesus Christ our Lord. These mortal bodies we inhabit are bent toward sin. Our hope and our salvation are in Christ and Christ alone.

Today's Scripture: *"When the perishable has been clothed with the imperishable, and the mortal with immortality, then the saying that is written will come true: 'Death has been swallowed up in victory'"* (1 Corinthians 15:54).

"But you have come to Mount Zion, to the heavenly Jerusalem, the city of the living God. You have come to thousands upon thousands of angels in joyful assembly, to the church of the firstborn, whose names are written in heaven. You have come to God, the judge of all men, to the spirits of righteous men made perfect" (Hebrews 12:22-23).

"But we have this treasure in jars of clay to show that this all-surpassing power is from God and not from us. We are hard pressed on every side, but not crushed; perplexed, but not in despair; persecuted, but not abandoned; struck down, but not destroyed. We always carry around in our body the death of Jesus, so that the life of Jesus may also be revealed in our body. For we who are alive are always being given over to death for Jesus' sake, so that his life may be revealed in our mortal body. So then, death is at work in us, but life is at work in you" (2 Corinthians 4:7-12).

Chapter 11

Question and Answers

$\mathcal{W}$hen my mother was first diagnosed with Alzheimer's disease, friends who had been in similar situations stepped forward to offer us prayer and support. Like a bucket brigade formed to quench fires of grief and fear, loving hands passed to us the knowledge they had gained during their own struggles with this disease. I have become a member of the brigade, and it has been my privilege to be able to help others toward solutions to their own challenges as they cope with the slow loss of a loved one. Here are some of the questions I have been asked, and I share answers from my own perspective and experience. Every situation is unique, and this is not meant to be a guide for other families. Seek out expert help.

Q: What factors caused you to choose to have your mother come to live with you rather than to place her in an assisted living situation or a rest home?

A: We truly had an unusual set of circumstances. I am an only child, and so the decision could be made quickly, without the collaboration that is appropriate when several families are affected by any decision that is made. My father had left a retirement fund that was just the right amount to pay for building an addition onto our home so that Mom could have a space of her own, affording our family a degree of privacy. My mother was not delusional or paranoid, and she handed over her finances to me with an attitude that changed quickly from trepidation to relief. She disliked physical exercise and so was not prone to wander away. Her income was adequate to allow her to pay me a small salary to care for her, and this in turn allowed me to cut my teaching job to half time without financial strain. We had not planned for these circumstances, beyond the fact that my father had been diligent to save money from each of his hard-earned paychecks. I always want to emphasize the fact that the term "caregiver" applies to any individual who feels ties of love and responsibility toward an individual who is infirm. The daughter who visits her mother weekly and manages her mom's finances is a caregiver. The son who lives across the country but calls the rest home frequently to ask for reports on a parent's condition is a caregiver. Every situation is unique, but God is Sovereign over them all.

Q: Does your mother have long term care insurance?

A: No. Mother did not apply for long term care insurance until she was seventy-seven years old, and then she was turned down. The long term care policies we researched would have paid for three years in a rest home. Some had provision for payment for in-home care. You have to find a good insurance agent and read the fine print.

Q: What was the sequence of actions you took when you suspected your mother was ill?

A: 1. I requested prayer from our pastor and from several trusted friends.

2. We visited our physician. Several tests were necessary to rule out other causes of dementia.

3. My mother began treatment with two medications designed specifically to treat Alzheimer's disease. Alzheimer's and depression often go hand in hand, and Mom benefited greatly from a prescription anti-depressant as well. She receives these three medications plus a few

vitamins and nutritional supplements daily. Information about Alzheimer's medications is easy to obtain online, at your library, or from the Alzheimer's Association. Do your homework and see your doctor. My mother experienced great improvement after initial treatment was begun and has maintained that higher level of functioning for over four years at this writing.

4. I received the benefit of guidance from friends who have faced similar situations.

5. I attended several meetings of our local chapter of the Alzheimer's Association, including one session called, "The ABC's of Alzheimer's Care."

6. We visited a lawyer who is an elder law expert. She was so helpful to us. With her knowledge we were able to make our plans to care for Mother ourselves in a way that would satisfy Medicaid's requirements in the case of a spend-down of Mother's assets once rest home care becomes necessary.

7. I obtained durable power of attorney for health care and financial decisions for my mother. This is a legal process and requires an attorney. It is vital for you to be able to make decisions for your loved ones at the point at which they can no longer decide for themselves.

8. We purchased a prepaid burial plan. This needed to be done because of the possibility that it would become necessary to "spend down" Mother's estate for rest home care, should she require it. I've since read that great caution is needed when purchasing prepaid plans and that there are other ways of putting money aside for this need that may be more prudent. Consult your lawyer with this concern. We live in a small town and our funeral director is a former Christian Youth Fellowship student of my Mom's. I'm comfortable with our solution.

Q: Is there anything you wish you had done differently?

A: Oh, of course. The mistakes I regret most came from the difficulty I had in adjusting my expectations of Mom in order to accommodate her decreasing level of functioning. For example, when she was first diagnosed, I somehow thought she could self-administer her medications, if only I would sort them into day of the week containers for her. Of course, she could not. She was ashamed, and she hid the pills from me. I wish that incidents such as this had not made me angry, and I wish I had not scolded her as though she were a child.

When a loved one is diagnosed with Alzheimer's disease we are given the facts. We learn that personality changes will occur. Paranoia, a self-centered perspective, and temper outbursts are all listed as possible symptoms as the disease progresses. On the part of a caregiver who is a close relative of the patient, there is an intellectual understanding of these facts; but it is difficult to transfer that "in the head" understanding to the heart. The tendency is to respond to the loved one based on the relationship that existed before dementia occurred. The caregiver must learn to respond to negative behaviors from a clinical and not an emotional perspective. It is a difficult transition, made easier by the recognition that although the rules of the relationship change, love remains.

And of course, any trial is made more difficult when we give way to fear. God always has a plan. If I could relive the past few years with more trust and less fear, everyone would benefit!

Q: What has been the biggest challenge of having your mother in your home?

A: By far the biggest challenge I've faced thus far is the emotional trauma of becoming my caregiver's caregiver! I've written about this transition throughout this book, but I must reemphasize the fact that if this transition is not acknowledged and prayed through, resentment and emotional detachment will result.

Q: Would you follow this same path again?

A: Absolutely, because this path was engineered for us by the Lord. I am so grateful to God for His power, His presence, and His provision for us during this time.

Endnotes

1   Taken from *My Utmost for His Highest*, by Oswald Chambers edited by James Reimann, August 29 devotion, *The Unsurpassed Intimacy of Tested Faith*, ©1992 by Oswald Chambers Publications Association, Ltd., and used by permission of Discovery House Publishers, Grand Rapids, MI 49501. All rights reserved.

2   *The Voyage of the Dawn Treader* by C.S.Lewis copyright © C.S. Lewis Pte. Ltd. 1952

3   Taken from *My Utmost for His Highest* by Oswald Chambers, edited by James Reimann, June 13 deovotion, *The Price of the Vision* © 1992 by Oswald Chambers Publications Association, Ltd., and used by permission of Discovery House Publishers, Grand Rapids, MI 49501. All rights reserved.

4   *What a Friend We Have in Jesus.* Music by: Charles Crozat Converse, 1868. Words by: Joseph Medlicott Scriven, 1885. This hymn is in public domain.

5   The Alzheimer's Association's brain tour at http://www.alz.org/brain/overview.asp Permission to cite granted via email.

6   Taken from *My Utmost for His Highest* by Oswald Chambers, edited by James Reimann, September 10 devotion, *Missionary Weapons*, © 1992 by Oswald Chambers Publications Association, Ltd., and used by permission of Discovery House Publishers, Grand Rapids, MI 49501 All rights reserved.

7   Taken from *The God of All Comfort* by Hannah Whitall Smith, this book is in public domain.

8   Hannah Whitall Smith's work is in public domain and can be accessed at the Christian Classics Ethereal Library online at http://www.ccel.org/

9   Taken from *My Utmost for His Highest* by Oswald Chambers, edited by James Reimann, August 2 devotion, *The Teaching of Adversity,* © 1992 by Oswald Chambers Publications Association, Ltd., and used by permission of Discovery House Publishers, Grand Rapids, MI 49501

10   *Immortal, Invisible, God Only Wise.* Words by Walter C Smith, 1876. Music by: St. Denio, Welsh Melody. This hymn is in public domain.

11   *The ABC's of Alzheimer's Care.* Reprinted with permission from the Alzheimer's Association of Northern California and Northern Nevada.

12   Poem, *What God Hath Promised* by Annie Johnson Flint. Public domain.

13   Chapter 7, Day 4, is about Sandy Smith. Permission to use this story was granted via an email dated January 29, 2007.

14   Chapter 7, Day 5, is about John and Amy Jarvis. Permission to use this story granted via an email dated February 7, 2007.

15   *Memory Matters Newsletter* published quarterly by the Alzheimer's Association—Heart of America Chapter. January, February, March 2007. *One Disease—Several Means of Support.*

16   This quote from John Piper was taken from *Decision* magazine, April 2006; © 2006 Billy Graham Evangelistic Association; used by permission, all rights reserved.

17   Taken from My Utmost for His Highest by Oswald Chambers, edited by James Reimann, June 18 devotion, Keep Recognizing Jesus © 1992 by Oswald Chambers Publications Association, LTD., and used by permission of Discovery House Publishers, Grand Rapids, MI 49501. All rights reserved.

18   Taken from *My Utmost for His Highest* by Oswald Chambers, edited by James Reimann, June 5 devotion, *God's Assurance* © 1992 by Oswald Chambers Publications Association, Ltd., and used by permission of Discovery House Publishers, Grand Rapids, MI 49501. All rights reserved.

19 Permission to quote granted by Reverend Warren Wilson via email March 17, 2007.

20 Quote taken from *Matthew Henry's Complete Commentary*. Public Domain

21 Taken from *My Utmost for His Highest* by Oswald Chambers, edited by James Reimann, February 25 devotion, *The Destitution of Service*, © 1992 by Oswald Chambers Publications Association, Ltd., and used by permission of Discovery House Publishers, Grand Rapids, MI 49501. All rights reserved.

Additonal readings for caregivers, contact information, and devotions for Alzheimer patients are available at Linda A. Born's web site http://www.godmomandme.com